ROSS & WILSON
Pocket Reference Guide to
Anatomy and Physiology

Anne Muller
Nurse, Senior Health Executive, Doctor of Educational Sciences and Instructor at the Health Management Training Institute, Ile-de-France, France

Translator and English Language Editor
Louis H. Honoré BSc(Hons) Physiology MBChB FRCPC LMCC
Professor Emeritus of Pathology, University of Alberta, Edmonton, Alberta, Canada

Foreword by
Anne Waugh BSc (Hons) MSc CertEd SRN RNT PFHEA
Former Senior Teaching Fellow and Senior Lecturer, School of Health and Social Care, Edinburgh Napier University, Edinburgh, UK
Allison Grant BSc PhD FHEA
Lecturer, Department of Health and Life Sciences, Glasgow Caledonian University, Glasgow, UK

ELSEVIER
Edinburgh   London   New York   Oxford   Philadelphia   St Louis   Sydney   2019

ELSEVIER

Anatomie et physiologie en fiches pour les étudiants en IFSI by Muller

© 2017, Elsevier Masson SAS. All rights reserved.

ISBN : 978-2-294-74849-3

This edition of *Anatomie et physiologie en fiches pour les étudiants en IFSI* by **Anne Muller** is published by arrangement with Elsevier Masson SAS.

Ross & Wilson Pocket Reference Guide to Anatomy and Physiology, First Edition

© 2019, Elsevier Limited. All rights reserved.

ISBN 978-0-7020-7617-6

Notices

Practitioners and researchers must always rely on their own experience and knowledge in evaluating and using any information, methods, compounds or experiments described herein. Because of rapid advances in the medical sciences, in particular, independent verification of diagnoses and drug dosages should be made. To the fullest extent of the law, no responsibility is assumed by Elsevier, authors, editors or contributors for any injury and/or damage to persons or property as a matter of products liability, negligence or otherwise, or from any use or operation of any methods, products, instructions, or ideas contained in the material herein.

Working together
to grow libraries in
developing countries

www.elsevier.com • www.bookaid.org

Content Strategist: Alison Taylor
Content Development Specialist: Kirsty Guest
Project Manager: Louisa Talbott
Design: Christian Bilbow
Illustration Manager: Teresa McBryan
Illustrator: Paula Catalano
Marketing Manager: Megan Richter

Printed in China

Last digit is the print number: 9 8 7 6 5 4 3 2 1

ROSS & WILSON

Pocket Reference Guide to
Anatomy and **Physiology**

Evolve®

YOU'VE JUST PURCHASED
MORE THAN
A TEXTBOOK!

Evolve Student Resources for *Muller: Ross & Wilson Pocket Reference Guide to Anatomy and Physiology, 1st Edition*, include the following:

- 80 MCQs to aid recall and application of core information.
- 100 labelling exercises to assist readers with the memorisation of anatomical structures.

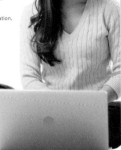

Activate the complete learning experience that comes with each textbook purchase by registering at

http://evolve.elsevier.com/Muller/

REGISTER TODAY!

ELSEVIER

2018v1.0

Key

Orientation compasses are used next to some of the figures, with paired directional terms above and below and on each side of the compass.

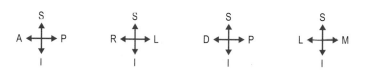

A/P: anterior–posterior. This indicates the relationship of the structure(s) to the front or back of the body (e.g. Fig. 19).

L/R: left–right (e.g. Fig. 1).

P/D: proximal–distal. This indicates the relationship of the structure(s) to the point of attachment to the body (e.g. Fig. 211).

L/M: lateral–medial. This indicates the relationship of the structure(s) to the midline of the body (e.g. Fig. 29).

S/I: superior–inferior. This indicates the relationship of the structure(s) to the upper or lower part of the body (e.g. Fig. 24).

Contents

Lymphatic system

Nervous system

Sense organs

Endocrine system

Respiratory system

The digestive system

Urinary system

The skin

Musculoskeletal system

The reproductive system

Foreword

This portable revision aid has been translated from a French volume by Anne Muller, and is designed to be a user-friendly, concise source of information. Its systematic, clear and well-illustrated content is drawn from the best-selling *Ross and Wilson Anatomy and Physiology in Health and Illness* publications, although it can also be used as a stand-alone resource to complement alternative textbooks. Whatever your anatomy and physiology learning needs are, we hope you find this book a convenient and helpful asset, and we wish you success in your studies.

Anne Waugh and Allison Grant
September 2018

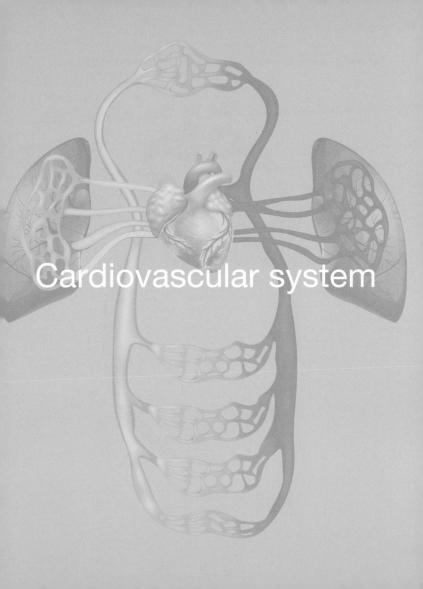

Cardiovascular system

The relationship between the pulmonary and systemic circulations

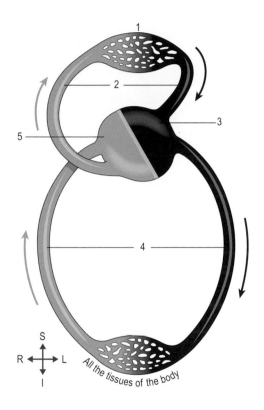

Fig 1

1. Lungs
2. Pulmonary system
3. Left side of the heart
4. Systemic circulation
5. Right side of the heart

Comments

Anatomical: There are two anatomically separate vascular systems. The pulmonary circulation—or the lesser circulation—carries blood from the right heart to the lungs and includes the pulmonary arteries and veins. The systemic circulation—or the greater circulation—carries blood from the left heart to the rest of the body and includes the aorta and its branches, as well as the venae cavae and their tributaries.

Physiological: The blood is the mode of transport of oxygen and carbon dioxide between the lungs and the cells of the body. In the lungs, where gas exchange occurs in the alveolar sacs, the blood extracts oxygen and releases carbon dioxide. The blood flowing to the organs of the body is rich in oxygen and nutrients, which are picked up by the cells of the body as they release their waste products into the blood for excretion.

Clinical: The arterial systolic pressure is higher in the systemic circulation. The colour of the skin and of the nails, whether pink or blue, reflects the functional state of the vascular and respiratory systems.

The inner aspect of a vein

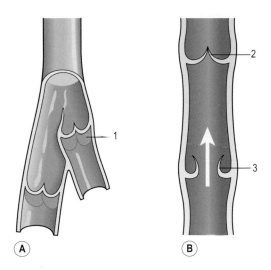

Fig 2 (A) The valves and the cusps. **(B)** The direction of blood flow through the valves.

1. Cusp
2. Cusp in closed position
3. Cusp in open position

Comments

Anatomical: The veins and arteries are made up of the same three tissue layers; the venous wall, however, is thinner because it contains fewer muscular and elastic fibres. The veins carry blood towards the heart. The insides of some veins contain semilunar valvular cusps, with their cavities pointing towards the heart to prevent any venous reflux.

Physiological: The veins allow the vascular system to adapt to changes in blood volume. If the volume increases, the veins, being capacitance vessels, dilate to increase the volume of blood being transported. If the blood volume decreases, they contract to prevent a fall in arterial pressure. The valves and their cusps inside the veins prevent venous reflux from happening. The veins collapse down when they are cut.

Clinical: The volume of blood in the veins amounts to two-thirds of the blood in the body. The cusps are numerous in the veins of the lower limbs but are not seen in the large veins of the thorax and of the abdomen, or in the venules. Dilated and tortuous veins indicate a build up of blood resulting from a slowing of the venous return. Varicosities, associated with pain and fatigue felt in the legs, are often seen in the saphenous and tibial veins.

The location of the heart in the thorax

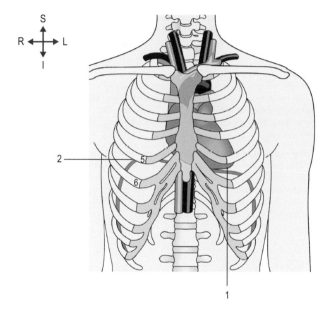

Fig 3

1. Apex of the heart in the fifth intercostal space, 9 cm from the median plane
2. The diaphragm at the level of the eighth thoracic vertebra

Comments

Anatomical: The region of the heart is demarcated by the lungs, the trachea and the large blood vessels. The heart, a hollow conical muscular organ, about 10 cm in length, is intrathoracic, lying within the mediastinum, which is the space between the two lungs. It is located towards the left side and the front of the body, with its pointed apex lying inferiorly in the fifth intercostal space and its base at the level of the second rib.

Physiological: The heart is responsible for supplying the whole body with blood.

Clinical: A man's heart is heavier than a woman's (310 g vs. 225 g). Anatomically locating the ribs helps position the electrodes efficiently during electrocardiography. The location of the heart explains the location of cardiac pain, which is thoracic for angina pectoris or myocardial infarction, with possible extension into the left arm and the jaw. This pain is transmitted by the T2 nerve, which arises at the level of the second thoracic vertebra and supplies a part of the arm and the skin of the axillary fossa.

Organs in relation to the heart

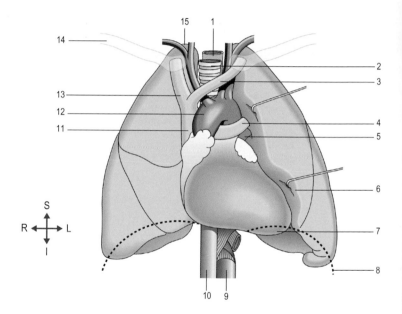

Fig 4

1. Oesophagus
2. Trachea
3. Left brachiocephalic vein
4. Pulmonary artery
5. Left pulmonary vein
6. Left lung (retracted)
7. Cardiac apex
8. Diaphragm
9. Aorta
10. Inferior vena cava
11. Superior vena cava
12. Aorta
13. Right brachiocephalic vein
14. Clavicle
15. Pulmonary apex

Comments

Anatomical: The heart lies obliquely more towards the left in the mediastinum. Its relations with the adjacent organs include the following:

a. *Posteriorly*—the trachea and the oesophagus, the main right and left bronchi, the descending aorta, the inferior vena cava and the thoracic vertebrae
b. *Anteriorly*—the sternum, the ribs and the intercostal muscles
c. *Laterally*—the lungs
d. *Superiorly*—the large vessels, the aorta, the superior vena cava, the pulmonary artery and the pulmonary veins
e. *Inferiorly*—the apex of the heart, supported by the central tendon of the diaphragm at the level of the fifth intercostal space

Physiological: The superior and inferior venae cavae drain into the right atrium. The blood then flows into the right ventricle and is propelled into the pulmonary trunk. The pulmonary veins return the oxygenated blood into the left atrium, from where it is conveyed into the left ventricle, across the mitral valve, before being ejected into the aorta.

Clinical: The pain due to pericarditis is thoracic and is exacerbated during deep breathing. The heart rate varies normally from person to person but can also vary as a result of disease. The heart rate is calculated as the number of cardiac beats per minute. An abnormally slow pulse is called *bradycardia*; an abnormally fast pulse is called *tachycardia*.

Layers of the wall of the heart

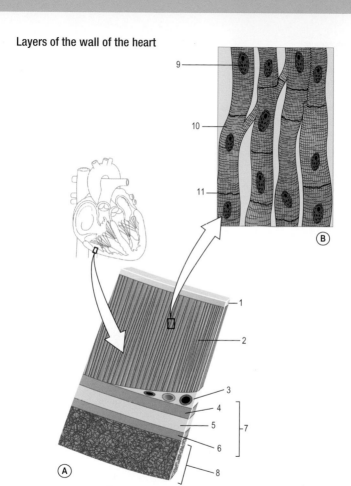

Fig 5 (A) Layers of the cardiac wall: endocardium, myocardium and pericardium.
(B) Heart muscle.

1. Endocardium
2. Myocardium
3. Fatty tissue and coronary vessels
4. Visceral pericardium
5. Pericardial space with pericardial fluid
6. Parietal pericardium
7. Serous pericardium
8. Fibrous pericardium
9. Nucleus
10. Branching cell
11. Intercalated disc

Comments

Anatomical: Three tissue layers make up the wall of the heart—the pericardium, the myocardium and the endocardium. The pericardium is the outer layer, consisting of two sacs, the outer one being the fibrous pericardium and the inner one being the serous pericardium. The fibrous pericardium is adherent to the diaphragm. Its nonelastic fibres restrict any excessive distention of the heart. The serous pericardium is made up of two layers, the parietal pericardium carpeting the fibrous pericardium and the visceral pericardium adherent to the cardiac muscle. The myocardium is a striated muscle tissue that specifically escapes voluntary control. Each myocardial fibre contains a nucleus and multiple branches. The cells are branched at their ends and form functional complexes, such as the partition-like intercalated discs. The myocardium is thicker at the apex at the level of the left ventricle. The endocardium, a thin and smooth membrane, covers the myocardium and the cardiac valves.

Physiological: The branches and the intercalated discs allow the electrical impulses to propagate and the cardiac muscle to contract as a syncytium. The contraction of the atria and of the ventricles is coordinated because of the sheet-like arrangement of the myocardium. A network of conducting fibres transmits the electrical signals to the heart muscle. The endocardium allows the blood to flow through the heart.

Clinical: Any irregular transmission of the electrical impulse and any slowing or speeding up of its transmission reflect conduction disturbances. Bradycardia can be a sign of an atrioventricular block and tachycardia a sign of atrial extrasystoles.

Inner aspect of the heart

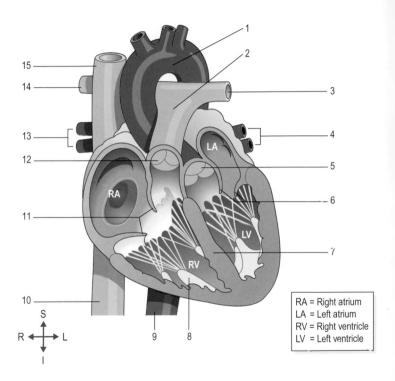

RA = Right atrium
LA = Left atrium
RV = Right ventricle
LV = Left ventricle

Fig 6

1. Aortic arch
2. Pulmonary trunk
3. Left pulmonary artery
4. Left pulmonary veins
5. Aortic valve
6. Mitral valve
7. Septum
8. Papillary muscle with chordae tendineae
9. Aorta
10. Inferior vena cava
11. Tricuspid valve
12. Pulmonary valve
13. Right pulmonary veins
14. Right pulmonary artery
15. Superior vena cava

Comments

Anatomical: The heart is divided by the cardiac septum into two parts, right and left. Each part is separated by an atrioventricular valve into an atrium and a ventricle. Derived from the endocardium, each valve contains cusps, three for the tricuspid and two for the mitral valves. The atrial myocardium is thinner than the ventricular myocardium. The pulmonary trunk arises from the upper part of the right ventricle, and the aorta arises from the upper part of the left ventricle.

Physiological: Blood flows from the atria towards the ventricles. The atria propel the blood towards the ventricles through the atrioventricular valves. The more powerful right and left ventricles expel the blood into the lungs and the rest of the body, respectively.

Clinical: After birth, the blood cannot move from the right to the left side of the heart via the septum. Blood moving to and fro between the two sides is abnormal.

The left mitral valve

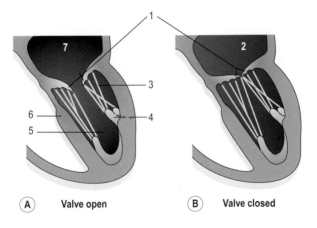

(A) Valve open

(B) Valve closed

Fig 7

1. Mitral valve (left atrioventricular valve)
2. Atrium
3. Chordae tendineae
4. Papillary muscle
5. Ventricle
6. Septum
7. Atrium

Comments

Anatomical: The mitral valve has two cusps. It is kept in place by the chordae tendineae, running from its internal aspect to the papillary muscles, which are structures derived from the myocardium and covered by endothelium.

Physiological: Blood flows from the atrium towards the ventricle. The mitral valve opens between the atrium and the ventricle when the pressure in the atrium is greater than that in the ventricle. It closes passively during ventricular contraction or ventricular systole, when the intraventricular pressure exceeds the intraatrial pressure. Its closure prevents reflux from ventricle into atrium.

Clinical: Reflux into the atrium during systole is due to malfunctioning of the mitral valve, such as mitral regurgitation.

Direction of blood flow inside the heart

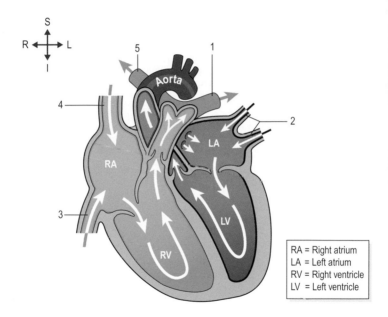

Fig 8

1. Left pulmonary artery
2. Left pulmonary veins
3. Inferior vena cava
4. Superior vena cava
5. Right pulmonary artery

Comments

Anatomical: The pulmonary and aortic valves are formed by three semilunar cusps.

Physiological: Blood transported by the inferior and superior venae cavae enters the right atrium, crosses the tricuspid valve and flows into the right ventricle, which propels it into the pulmonary trunk across the pulmonary valve. This then prevents reflux of blood from the pulmonary trunk into the ventricle when the latter relaxes. The pulmonary trunk divides into two branches, the right and the left, which carry venous blood into the lungs, where there is gas exchange of oxygen and carbon dioxide. The oxygen is absorbed, and the carbon dioxide is excreted. Two pulmonary veins carry the oxygenated blood from each lung into the left atrium; there are four pulmonary veins involved. The blood crosses the mitral valve to enter the left ventricle, from where it is ejected into the aorta.

Clinical: Pulmonary oedema and oedema of the lower limbs can indicate a valvulopathy or valvular malfunction due to defective opening or closing of the valve. The aortic and mitral valves are the two valves that are most frequently involved.

Section of the aorta opened to show the semilunar cusps of the aortic valve

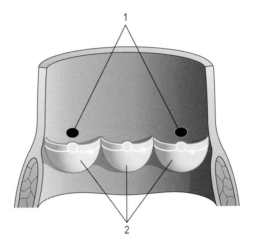

Fig 9

1. Orifices of the right and left coronary arteries
2. Semilunar cusps

Comments

Anatomical: The aortic valve is a cardiac valve, an anatomical structure separating the ventricle from the aorta. It is made up of three semilunar cusps – one dorsal, one anterolateral on the left and one anterolateral on the right. Above these cusps arise the coronary arteries, which supply the cardiac muscle with blood.

Physiological: The semilunar cusps prevent reflux of blood into the left ventricle. During systole, the blood-filled ventricle contracts and ejects its contents into the aorta across the aortic valve to supply the organs with blood. During diastole, the aortic valve is closed. Its opening and closure are passive, depending on the pressure difference on either side of the valve. It opens when the pressure downstream is less than the pressure upstream; it closes when the pressures are reversed.

Clinical: Normally, the arterial pressure is less than 140/90 mmHg. The first number is the systolic pressure (the pressure associated with systole) and the second is the diastolic pressure (the pressure associated with diastole). Closure of the aortic valve corresponds to the second heart sound on cardiac auscultation; the first heart sound corresponds to the closure of the mitral and tricuspid valves. Shortness of breath made worse by lying down or by physical exertion, fatigue, a feeling of heavy discomfort in the chest, palpitations, bilateral ankle oedema and weight gain are signs of an anatomical lesion or malfunction of the valve.

The flow of blood inside the heart and the systemic and pulmonary circulations

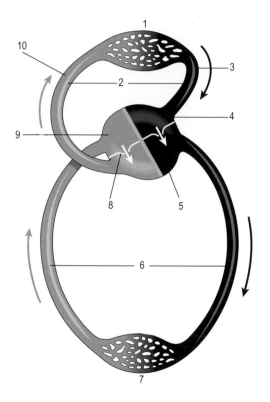

Fig 10

1. Lungs
2. Pulmonary circulation
3. Pulmonary vein
4. Left side of the heart
5. Mitral valve
6. Systemic circulation
7. All the body tissues
8. Tricuspid valve
9. Right side of the heart
10. Pulmonary artery

Comments

Physiological: The systemic circulation propels blood from the left heart to and from the organs of the body via the aorta and its branches and the venae cavae and their collaterals. The aorta arises from the heart, carries blood rich in oxygen and poor in carbon dioxide to all the organs of the body and then ensures return of the blood, now poor in oxygen and rich in carbon dioxide, to the heart via the superior and inferior venae cavae. The blood flows from the right side to the left side of the heart via the pulmonary circulation, which conveys the blood from the right heart through the lungs in the pulmonary arteries and veins. The pulmonary trunk carries the venous blood poor in oxygen and rich in carbon dioxide to the pulmonary alveoli for reoxygenation and ensures its return to the heart via the pulmonary veins.

Clinical: Arterial hypotension occurs when the systolic pressure is below 100 mmHg. When a person stands up rapidly from a lying down or sitting position, this change of position can cause a drop in blood pressure known as *orthostatic arterial hypotension*. Obesity, pyrexia, physical activity, emotion and some diseases may cause hypertension, which may be transient. Persistent hypertension wears out the heart.

The coronary arteries

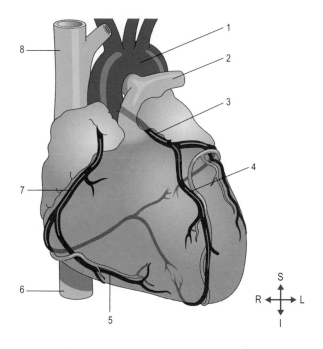

Fig 11

1. Aortic arch
2. Pulmonary artery
3. Left coronary artery
4. Branch of the left coronary artery
5. Branch of the right coronary artery
6. Inferior vena cava
7. Right coronary artery
8. Superior vena cava

Comments

Anatomical: The heart receives blood via the right and left coronary arteries, which arise from the aorta just above the aortic valve. They receive about 5% of the blood ejected by the aorta during each systole. They penetrate the wall of the heart and form a network of capillaries. The right and left coronary arteries divide into branches.

Physiological: The coronary arteries and their branches supply the cardiac muscle with the blood coming from the aorta.

Clinical: Inadequate blood supply to the myocardium, mostly due to coronary atherosclerosis, is called *coronary artery disease*. Its clinical signs and symptoms include discomfort or pain in the left chest (angina pectoris), with or without spread to the shoulder or arm, difficulty in breathing and extreme fatigue on exertion.

The conducting system of the heart

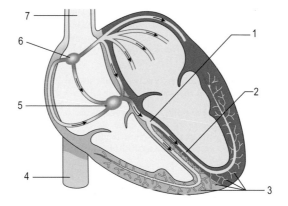

Fig 12

1. Atrioventricular bundle
2. Left bundle branch of atrioventricular bundle
3. Network of Purkinje fibres
4. Inferior vena cava
5. Atrioventricular node
6. Sino-atrial node
7. Superior vena cava

Comments

Anatomical: The myocardium contains nodal or conducting tissue made up of groups of specialised muscle cells. The sinoatrial node is located in the wall of the right atrium, near the opening of the superior vena cava. The atrioventricular node lies near the atrioventricular valves. The Purkinje fibre network forms part of the atrioventricular bundle, which arises from the atrioventricular node.

Physiological: The heart is characterised by an inherent myogenic rhythm solely responsible for the heartbeat. The specialised muscle cells of the sinoatrial node initiate the impulses and organise and coordinate the contraction of the muscle cells. The myocardium is innervated by sympathetic and parasympathetic nerve fibres that increase or decrease the heart rate. The electrical impulse starts in the sinoatrial node, traverses the right and left atria and causes them to contract and propel the blood into the ventricles. From there on, it enters the ventricles via the atrioventricular node, travels along the atrioventricular bundle and sets off the contraction of the ventricle and the propulsion of the blood towards the lungs and the body.

Clinical: At rest, the heart rate is between 60 and 80 beats per minute. A heartbeat corresponds to a cardiac cycle comprised of one systole and one diastole. The heart first contracts and then relaxes. Any abnormality of the conduction system, whether it involves disturbances in rhythm or in the conduction process, can produce a heart rate that is too slow, too fast or irregular and constitutes a cardiac emergency.

The skeletal muscle pump

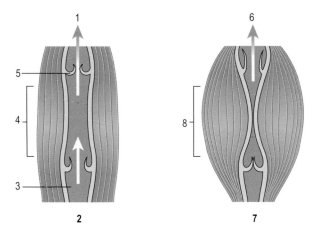

Fig 13

1. Towards the heart
2. Open valves
3. Vein
4. Muscle relaxed
5. Valve
6. Towards the heart
7. Proximal valve open; distal valve closed
8. Muscle contracted

Comments

Anatomical: The blood moves from the heart towards the organs and comes back from the organs to the heart.

Physiological: Venous return influences the cardiac output. The propulsive action of the left ventricle is inadequate to achieve this round trip movement of blood. Muscular contraction helps propel blood towards the heart by compressing the deep veins. The skeletal muscle pump results from this muscular activity taking place in the lower limbs. The venous valves prevent any reflux of the blood.

Clinical: Physical activity associated with muscular contraction facilitates venous return, unlike prolonged standing or sitting. The efficiency of venous return also requires an intact system of venous valves.

The main sites for taking the pulse

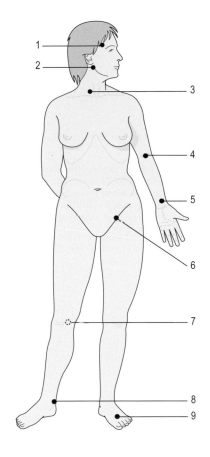

1
2
3
4
5
6
7
8
9

Fig 14

1. Temporal artery
2. Facial artery
3. Common carotid artery
4. Brachial artery
5. Radial artery
6. Femoral artery
7. Popliteal artery (behind the knee)
8. Posterior tibial artery
9. Dorsalis pedis artery

Comments

Physiological: Each contraction of the left ventricle propels 60 to 80 mL of blood into the aorta, which is distended. This distention is propagated as a wave that is carried along the walls of the arteries.

Clinical: This distention wave can be felt clinically when a superficial artery is pressed against a bone. The pulse is palpated by gently applying pressure on a superficial artery during ventricular systole, when the arterial wall is distended by the blood ejected from the left ventricle. It is due to the lifting of the arterial wall. The pulse frequency is equal to the number of heartbeats, except in cases of arrhythmia, when the heart rate is determined by auscultation of the heart, because some contractions are ineffectual and are not transmitted down to the distal arteries. The pulse varies from person to person. At rest, it ranges from 60 to 80 per minute. The pulse rate can be taken at different points on the body and provides information about the heart rate, the regularity and force of the beats and the tension exerted on the arterial wall. The pulse rate reflects the time interval between the heartbeats. This interval may or may not be the same. Tachycardia, bradycardia or any change in the cardiac rhythm is a sign of rhythm or conduction disturbances.

The aorta and the main arteries of the limbs

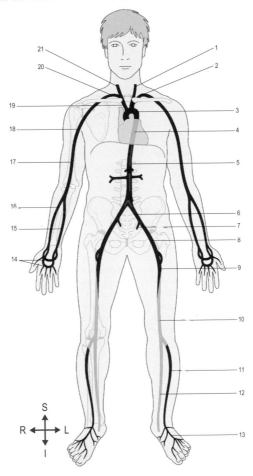

Fig 15

1. Left common carotid artery
2. Left subclavian artery
3. Aortic arch
4. Thoracic aorta
5. Abdominal aorta
6. Left common iliac artery
7. Left internal iliac artery
8. Left external iliac artery
9. Left femoral artery
10. Left popliteal artery
11. Left anterior tibial artery
12. Left posterior tibial artery
13. Dorsalis pedis artery
14. Right digital palmar arches
15. Right ulnar artery
16. Right radial artery
17. Right brachial artery
18. Right axillary artery
19. Brachiocephalic trunk
20. Right subclavian artery
21. Right common carotid artery

Comments

Anatomical: The aorta, the largest artery in the body, arises from the left ventricle and gives rise to the thoracic aorta (including the arch) and the abdominal aorta. It also gives rise to the arteries that supply the limbs. Some of its branches are paired, one on the right and the other on the left of the body.

Physiological: The blood is carried by the aorta and its branches from the heart to the whole of the body. This segment of the circulation is known as arterial.

Clinical: The pulse can be taken at the level of each of these arteries — temporal, facial, common carotid, brachial, radial, femoral, popliteal, posterior tibial and dorsalis pedis.

The venae cavae and the main veins of the limbs

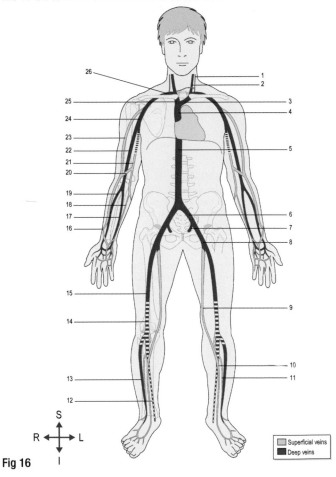

Fig 16

S
R ←→ L
I

Superficial veins
Deep veins

1. Left external jugular vein
2. Left internal jugular vein
3. Left brachiocephalic vein
4. Superior vena cava
5. Inferior vena cava
6. Left common iliac vein
7. Left internal iliac vein
8. Left external iliac vein
9. Left great saphenous vein
10. Left great saphenous vein
11. Left small saphenous vein
12. Right posterior tibial vein
13. Right anterior tibial vein
14. Right popliteal vein
15. Right femoral vein
16. Right cephalic vein
17. Right ulnar vein
18. Right median vein
19. Right radial vein
20. Right median cubital vein
21. Right basilic vein
22. Right brachial vein
23. Right cephalic vein
24. Right axillary vein
25. Right brachiocephalic vein
26. Right subclavian vein

Comments

Anatomical: The superior and inferior venae cavae are the two largest veins in the body. They arise from the fusion of different veins, some of which are paired, one on the left and the other on the right of the body.

Physiological: The superior and inferior venae cavae and their tributaries drain the blood coming, respectively, from above and from below the diaphragm and empty their contents into the right atrium. This segment of the circulation is known as the venous circulation.

Clinical: Venepuncture takes advantage of the abundance of veins. Thrombosis or thrombotic occlusion can occur anywhere in the venous system in certain pathological states.

The aorta and its main branches

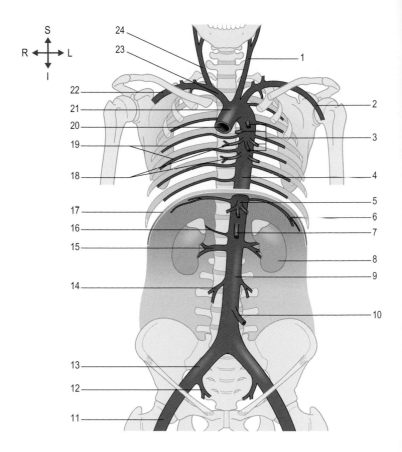

Fig 17

1. Left common carotid artery
2. Left subclavian artery
3. Bronchial arteries
4. Thoracic aorta
5. Coeliac trunk
6. Left inferior phrenic artery
7. Superior mesenteric artery
8. Left kidney
9. Abdominal aorta
10. Inferior mesenteric artery
11. Right external iliac artery
12. Right internal iliac artery
13. Right common iliac artery
14. Right ovarian/testicular artery
15. Right renal artery
16. Right suprarenal artery
17. Diaphragm
18. Oesophageal arteries
19. Intercostal arteries
20. Ascending aorta
21. Aortic arch
22. Right subclavian artery
23. Right brachiocephalic artery
24. Right common carotid artery

Comments

Anatomical: The aorta arises from the left ventricle and divides into many collateral branches. It curves to descend inside the thoracic cavity. The thoracic aorta has two collateral branches, the right and the left coronary arteries. The aorta crosses the aortic hiatus, passes under the diaphragm at the level of the 12th thoracic vertebra and then descends into the abdominal cavity, down to the level of the fourth lumbar vertebra. The abdominal aorta divides into the paired right and left common iliac arteries.

Physiological: The aorta is a large-bore artery that carries blood to all the organs, including the brain.

Clinical: The diameter of the abdominal aorta is about 2 cm. A diameter greater than 3 cm would raise the possibility of an aneurysm, which is an abnormal dilation of its wall. It is initially silent and then gives rise to the following symptoms: abdominal pain, a sense of heaviness and discomfort. A diameter exceeding 5 cm has a high risk of rupture, which can be fatal. An aneurysm can also occur in the thoracic aorta.

The venae cavae and their main tributaries

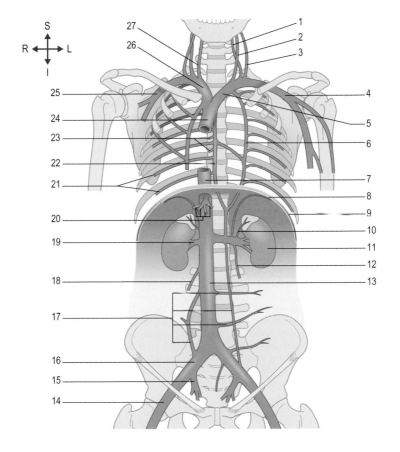

Fig 18

1. Vertebral vein
2. Left internal jugular vein
3. Left external jugular vein
4. Left subclavian vein
5. Left brachiocephalic vein
6. Hemiazygos vein
7. Inferior vena cava (thoracic part)
8. Phrenic vein
9. Diaphragm
10. Left suprarenal vein
11. Left kidney
12. Left ovarian/testicular vein
13. Inferior vena cava (abdominal part)
14. Right external iliac vein
15. Right internal iliac vein
16. Right common iliac vein
17. Lumbar veins
18. Right ovarian/testicular vein
19. Right renal vein
20. Hepatic veins
21. Intercostal veins
22. Azygos vein
23. Oesophageal veins
24. Superior vena cava
25. Right subclavian vein
26. Right brachiocephalic vein
27. Right internal jugular vein

Comments

Anatomical: The superior vena cava measures 7 cm in length.

Physiological: The superior and inferior venae cavae drain the venous blood from the entire body towards the heart. The right and left brachiocephalic veins join to form the superior vena cava, which drains into the right atrium. The veins coming from the pelvic and abdominal organs drain into the inferior vena cava, which arises from the fusion of the right and left common iliac veins at the level of the fifth lumbar vertebra. It ascends up the abdomen close to the vertebral column before entering the right atrium.

Clinical: Thrombosis can develop anywhere in the venous system in some diseases.

The main arteries of the left side of the head and neck

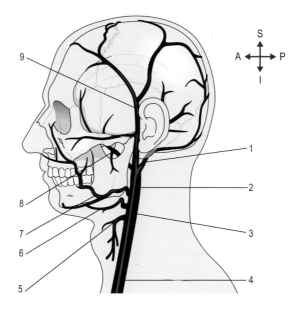

Fig 19

1. Occipital artery
2. External carotid artery
3. Internal carotid artery
4. Common carotid artery
5. Superior thyroid artery
6. Lingual artery
7. Facial artery
8. Maxillary artery
9. Superficial temporal artery

Comments

Anatomical: The left common carotid artery arises from the aortic arch and gives rise to the external and internal carotid arteries. The right common carotid artery arises from the brachiocephalic trunk.

Physiological: The arteries supplying the two sides of the head and neck are the common carotid and the vertebral arteries. The external carotid artery supplies the tissues of the head and neck with blood via its many branches the superficial temporal, the maxillary, the facial, the lingual, the superior thyroid and the occipital arteries. The internal carotid artery and its branches supply the forehead, the eye and the nose. The two internal carotid arteries and the two vertebral arteries form the arterial circle of Willis, which supplies most of the brain.

Clinical: Movements of the head and of the neck and blockage in one artery of the circle of Willis do not cut off the blood supply to the brain, which, on the other hand, can be affected by thrombotic events, usually involving the aortic arch and the carotid arteries.

The arteries forming the cerebral arterial circle (the circle of Willis) and its main branches to the brain (seen from below)

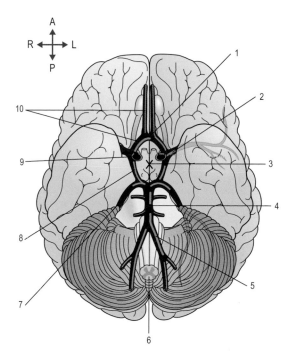

Fig 20

1. Anterior communicating artery
2. Left middle cerebral artery
3. Circle of Willis
4. Basilar artery
5. Left vertebral artery
6. Spinal cord
7. Right posterior cerebral artery
8. Right posterior communicating artery
9. Right internal carotid artery
10. Right anterior cerebral artery

Comments

Anatomical: The circle of Willis is formed by four arteries—the right and left carotid arteries and the right and left vertebral arteries, with the latter arising from the right and left subclavian arteries, respectively.

Physiological: The circle of Willis supplies most of the brain via 10 arteries—the two anterior cerebral arteries, the two posterior cerebral arteries, one anterior communicating artery in contrast to two posterior communicating arteries, two carotid arteries and one basilar artery. The vertebral arteries supply the brain, the internal carotid arteries supply the brain and the eyes, and the external carotid arteries supply the skin of the cranium and of the face.

Clinical: The circle of Willis is designed to supply the brain adequately. This arterial anastomotic system can offset the blockage of one artery. The brain can still receive blood rich in oxygen and nutrients, even if one of the neck arteries is damaged or blocked.

The right vertebral artery

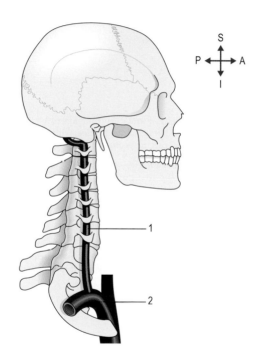

Fig 21

1. Right vertebral artery
2. Right subclavian artery

Comments

Anatomical: The right vertebral artery runs along the right side of the neck. After arising from the right subclavian artery, it ascends towards the foramen transversarium of the sixth cervical vertebra, goes through it and the following foramina transversaria of the fifth, fourth and third vertebrae to reach the atlas (the first cervical vertebra) and the medulla oblongata. The two vertebral arteries then unite to form the basilar artery.

Physiological: The vertebral artery supplies the posterior part of the brain and part of the spinal cord. The branches of the basilar artery supply part of the brain stem and the cerebellum. The basilar artery supplies the posterior cerebrum, the cerebellum and the brain stem (via the posteroinferior cerebellar artery and the basilar artery) and the spinal cord.

Clinical: Vertigo may be a sign of cerebellar vascular insufficiency, but this is not its most common cause.

The veins of the left side of the head and neck

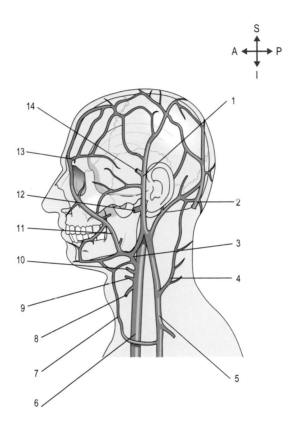

Fig 22

1. Left superficial temporal vein
2. Left occipital vein
3. Left common facial vein
4. Left external posterior jugular vein
5. Left external jugular vein
6. Left internal jugular vein
7. Left anterior jugular vein
8. Left superior thyroid vein
9. Left pharyngeal vein
10. Left lingual vein
11. Left facial vein
12. Left maxillary vein
13. Left supraorbital vein
14. Left middle temporal vein

Comments

Anatomical: The superficial veins—the superficial temporal, maxillary, facial, lingual, superior thyroid and occipital veins—unite to form the external jugular vein, which then drains into the subclavian vein. The external jugular vein starts at the angle of the mandible in the neck and joins the subclavian vein.

Physiological: Venous return from the head and neck is via the superficial and deep veins. The venous blood from the deep layers of the brain drains into the venous sinuses.

Clinical: Dilation or congestion of the jugular vein in the neck is a sign of right-sided cardiac failure, which can be associated with the hepatojugular reflux observed in the jugular vein when the abdomen is compressed by an examiner. The jugular vein can be used for blood transfusion.

The main arteries of the right arm

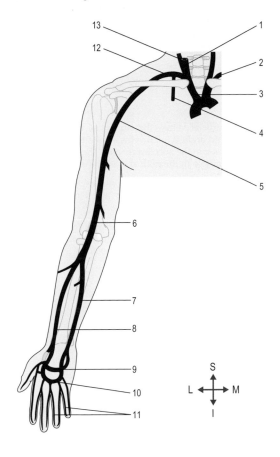

Fig 23

1. Right common carotid artery
2. Left subclavian artery
3. Brachiocephalic artery
4. Right internal thoracic artery
5. Right axillary artery
6. Right brachial artery
7. Right ulnar artery

8. Right radial artery
9. Right deep palmar arch
10. Right superficial palmar arch
11. Right digital arteries
12. Right subclavian artery
13. Right vertebral artery

Comments

Anatomical: The upper limb is supplied by the ipsilateral subclavian artery. The right subclavian artery, arising from the brachiocephalic trunk, becomes continuous with the axillary artery and then with the brachial, radial and ulnar arteries. The axillary artery passes under the clavicle in the axilla. The radial and ulnar arteries anastomose to form the superficial and deep palmar arterial arches, which give rise to the digital arteries.

Physiological: The right subclavian artery and its branches supply the right upper limb.

Clinical: The pulse can be palpated at the level of the radial and brachial arteries. An arterial catheter inserted into the radial artery allows the arterial blood pressure to be monitored continuously and blood samples to be taken, without the need to keep pricking the patient repeatedly.

The main veins of the right arm

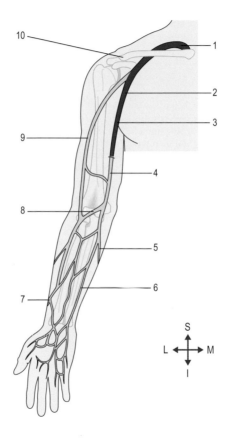

Fig 24

1. Right subclavian vein
2. Right axillary vein
3. Right brachial vein
4. Right basilic vein
5. Right basilic vein
6. Right median vein
7. Right cephalic vein
8. Right median cubital vein
9. Right cephalic vein
10. Right clavicle

Comments

Anatomical: The cephalic vein receives the venous blood from the superficial veins of the dorsum of the hand.

Physiological: The venous return from the right upper limb occurs in the deep veins (the subclavian, axillary, brachial, radial and ulnar veins, the deep palmar venous arch and the palmar metacarpal veins) and in the superficial veins (the cephalic, basilic, median and median cubital veins). The internal jugular vein joins the subclavian, which carries the blood from the upper limb to form the brachiocephalic vein before draining into the superior vena cava.

The coeliac artery with its branches

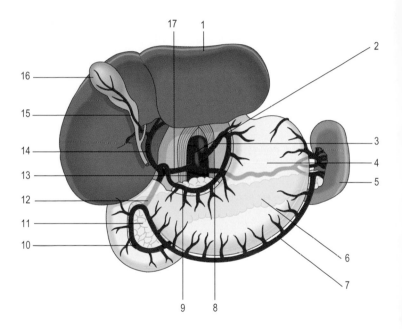

Fig 25

1. Liver (raised)
2. Coeliac artery
3. Left gastric artery
4. Stomach
5. Spleen
6. Pancreas
7. Left gastroepiploic artery
8. Splenic artery
9. Hight gastric artery
10. Right gastroepiploic artery
11. Head of pancreas
12. Gastroduodenal artery
13. Aorta
14. Right hepatic artery
15. Cystic artery
16. Gall bladder
17. Common hepatic artery

Comments

Anatomical: The coeliac artery, also called the *coeliac trunk*, springs from the aorta below the diaphragm; it measures about 1.25 cm in length.

Physiological: It divides into three branches, which supply the following abdominal organs: the left gastric artery for the stomach, the splenic artery for the pancreas and spleen and the common hepatic artery for the liver, the gall bladder, the pancreas, the stomach and the duodenum.

The superior and inferior mesenteric arteries and their branches

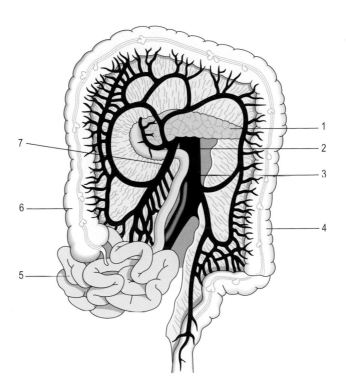

Fig 26

1. Pancreas
2. Aorta
3. Inferior mesenteric artery
4. Descending colon (part of the large intestine)
5. The small intestine (displaced)
6. Ascending colon (part of the large intestine)
7. Superior mesenteric artery

Comments

Anatomical: The superior and inferior mesenteric arteries arise from the abdominal aorta. The superior mesenteric artery arises at the level of the first lumbar vertebra at the same level as the renal artery. The inferior mesenteric artery arises at the level of the third lumbar vertebra.

Physiological: The superior mesenteric artery supplies the small intestine and the ascending colon. It gives off the following branches — the inferior pancreaticoduodenal artery, the right colic artery supplying the right colic flexure, the middle colic artery supplying the ascending colon and the ileocolic artery supplying the ileocaecal region. The inferior mesenteric artery supplies the descending colon and part of the rectum.

Clinical: The syndrome of abdominal pain after eating, known as *intestinal ischaemia,* can be due to narrowing of the superior mesenteric artery.

The venous drainage of the abdominal organs and the formation of the portal vein

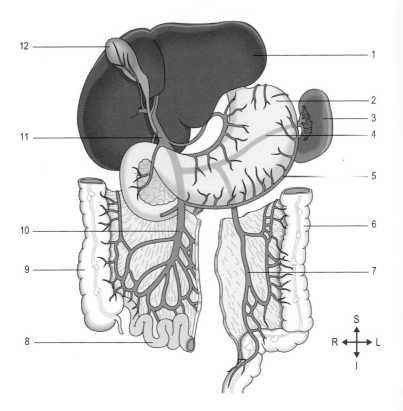

Fig 27

1. Liver
2. Stomach
3. Spleen
4. Splenic vein
5. Right gastroepiploic vein
6. Part of the large intestine
7. Inferior mesenteric vein
8. Part of the small intestine
9. Part of the large intestine
10. Superior mesenteric vein
11. Portal vein
12. Gall bladder

Comments

Anatomical: The portal vein arises from the fusion of multiple veins — the splenic, superior mesenteric, inferior mesenteric, gastric and cystic veins.

Physiological: The venous blood from the rectum, sigmoid colon and descending colon drains into the inferior mesenteric vein before it joins the splenic vein, which receives the venous drainage of the spleen, the pancreas and part of the stomach. Venous drainage of the small intestine, the ascending colon and the caecum occurs via the superior mesenteric vein. The gastric veins drain the venous blood from the stomach and the oesophagus; the cystic vein drains the venous blood from the gall bladder. The venous blood from these different veins drains into the portal vein and then into the hepatic veins before reaching the inferior vena cava.

The portal vein: its origin and termination

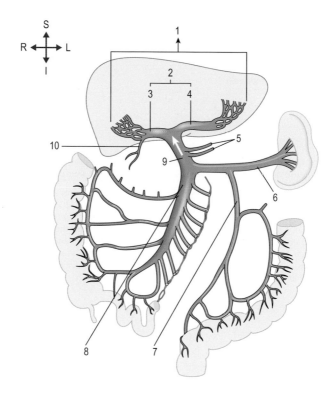

Fig 28

1. Flow towards the hepatic sinusoids
2. Portal vein
3. Right branch
4. Left branch
5. Gastric veins
6. Splenic vein
7. Inferior mesenteric vein
8. Superior mesenteric vein
9. Portal vein
10. Cystic vein

Comments

Anatomical: The splenic, superior mesenteric, inferior mesenteric, gastric and cystic veins converge to form the portal vein.

Physiological: The venous blood drains via these different veins to reach the portal vein, from where it enters the hepatic veins before draining into the inferior vena cava. Cirrhosis or a tumour of the liver can cause portal vein thrombosis.

The femoral artery and its main branches

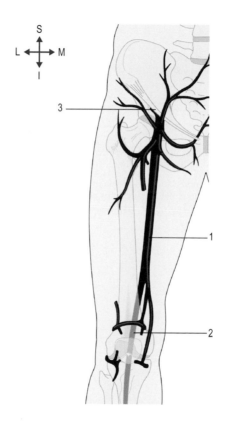

Fig 29

1. Femoral artery
2. Popliteal artery
3. Inguinal ligament

Comments

Anatomical: The right or left femoral artery arises from the ipsilateral external iliac artery deep to the inguinal ligament and, in the thigh, it splits into the deep and the superficial femoral arteries. At the knee, the superficial femoral artery turns into the popliteal artery, which then divides into three branches.

Physiological: The femoral artery supplies the structures of the thigh and the pelvic and inguinal regions of the body.

Clinical: The femoral pulse is taken at the origin of the femoral artery. This artery is at risk of developing atherosclerosis, which can cause lower limb ischaemia during walking initially and at rest in its more advanced stages. It can also give rise to an aneurysm, with the risk of rupture and haemorrhage.

The popliteal artery and its main branches

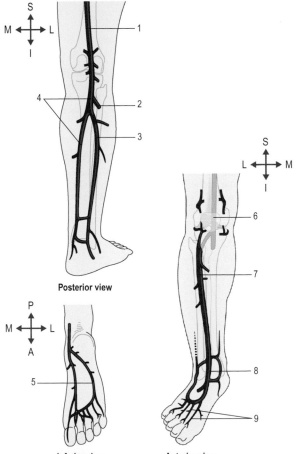

S
M ← → L
I

1

4
2
3

S
L ← → M
I

6

7

8

9

Posterior view

P
M ← → L
A

5

Inferior view

Anterior view

Fig 30

Posterior view
1. Popliteal artery
2. Anterior tibial artery
3. Fibular artery
4. Posterior tibial artery

Inferior view
5. Plantar arch

Anterior view
6. Popliteal artery
7. Anterior tibial artery
8. Dorsalis pedis artery
9. Digital arteries

Comments

Anatomical: The popliteal artery is the continuation of the femoral artery and divides into the anterior and posterior tibial arteries, which give rise to the dorsalis pedis and digital arteries. The posterior tibial artery also gives rise to the fibular artery, which becomes the plantar artery and the plantar arch.

Physiological: The popliteal artery supplies the popliteal fossa and the knee joint. The anterior tibial artery supplies the anterior aspect of the thigh. The plantar and the dorsalis pedis arteries supply the feet. The fibular artery supplies the lateral part of the thigh.

Clinical: The popliteal pulse is taken at the level of the popliteal fossa, behind the knee. Rupture of a popliteal aneurysm or damage to its wall can cause bleeding. The popliteal artery can also develop atherosclerosis, giving rise to ischaemic pain in the thigh or necrosis of the toes in severe cases.

The superficial veins of the lower limb

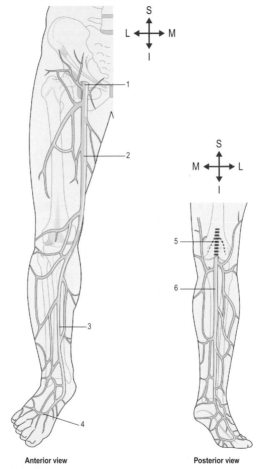

Fig 31   Anterior view   Posterior view

Anterior view
1. Femoral vein
2. Great saphenous vein
3. Great saphenous vein
4. Dorsal venous arch

Posterior view
5. Popliteal vein
6. Small saphenous vein

Comments

Physiological: The venous blood from the lower limb drains into two superficial veins, the small and the great saphenous veins. The small saphenous vein receives the venous blood from the dorsum of the foot and flows into the popliteal vein. The large saphenous vein joins the femoral vein deep to the inguinal ligament. The popliteal and the femoral veins are deep veins. The internal and external iliac veins join to form the common iliac veins, which in turn unite to form the inferior vena cava. There are communicating veins that run between the superficial veins themselves and also between the superficial and deep veins. The venous return to the heart depends on the contraction of the skeletal muscles and on the venous valves.

Clinical: The veins can become varicose, with damage to their walls, as a result of slowing or pooling of blood due to incompetence of the valves. The risk of thrombosis is related to the formation of an intravascular blood clot because of a lesion in the vessel wall or as a result of predisposing factors, such as immobilisation and prolonged confinement to bed.

The relationship of the placenta to the uterine wall

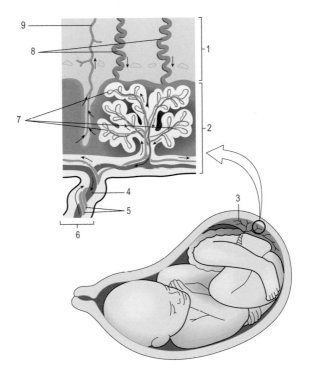

Fig 32

1. Endometrium
2. Placenta
3. Placenta
4. Umbilical vein
5. Umbilical arteries
6. Umbilical cord
7. Fetal capillaries bathed in maternal blood
8. Maternal arterioles
9. Maternal venule

Comments

Anatomical: The placenta develops from the fertilised ovum. It consists of fetal capillaries bathed in maternal blood. It is attached on the one side to the uterine wall and on the other to the fetus by the umbilical cord, which enters the fetus at the umbilicus. This cord is about 50 cm long. It contains two arteries and one vein. The placenta is expelled from the uterus after birth.

Physiological: The placenta is the seat of exchange of substances, nutrients and waste products between the separate circulatory systems of the mother and fetus. The umbilical arteries carry the poorly oxygenated blood from the fetus to the placenta, whereas the umbilical vein brings back well-oxygenated blood to the fetus. These exchanges take place at the level of the fetal capillaries, which are bathed in maternal blood. The fetal blood gets rid of carbon dioxide and waste products and picks up oxygen and nutrients. Maternal antibodies cross the placenta and thus help protect the fetus. The placenta has an endocrine function by secreting human chorionic gonadotropin (hCG) and oestrogen, hormones that protect and maintain the pregnancy.

Clinical: If the placental circulation is deficient—that is, if there is placental insufficiency—the fetus may show growth retardation associated with reduced body weight.

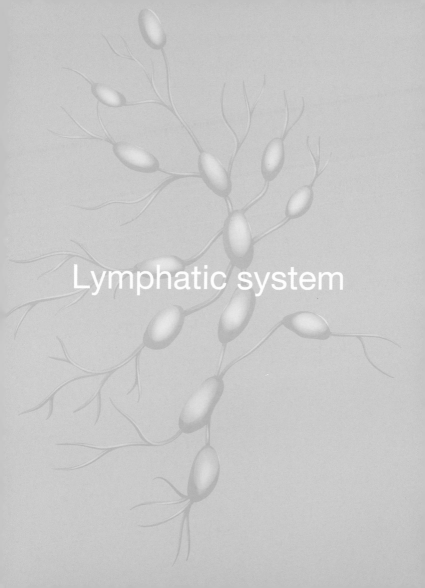

Lymphatic system

The main constituents of the lymphatic system

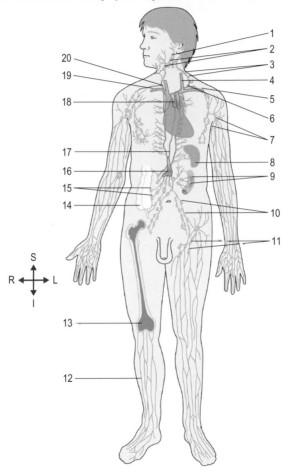

Fig 33

1. Palatine tonsil
2. Submandibular lymph nodes
3. Cervical lymph nodes
4. Left internal jugular vein
5. Left subclavian vein
6. Thoracic duct
7. Axillary lymph nodes
8. Spleen
9. Aggregate lymphoid nodules (Peyer's patches)
10. Small intestine
11. Inguinal lymph nodes
12. Lymphatic vessel
13. Red bone marrow
14. Large intestine
15. Intestinal lymph nodes
16. Cisterna chyli
17. Thoracic duct
18. Thymus
19. Right subclavian vein
20. Right lymphatic duct

Comments

Anatomical: The lymphatic system consists of lymph, vessels, nodes, lymphatic organs, lymphoid tissue and bone marrow. The lymph is carried by capillaries that join to form large lymphatic vessels that coalesce into two channels: (1) the thoracic duct; and (2) the right lymphatic duct. The first drains the lymph from the lower limbs, the pelvic and abdominal cavities, the left half of the head and neck and the left upper limb. It arises from the cisterna chyli, crosses the abdomen and the thorax and then joins the left subclavian vein. The second drains the lymph from the right half of the thorax and of the head and neck and of the right upper limb. The lymph nodes, arranged as deep and superficial nodes along the lymphatic vessels of the body, receive and filter lymph. The lymphoid tissue resides in lymphatic organs such as the spleen and the thymus; it is also disseminated in multiple sites, such as the tonsils, the mouth and the aggregate lymphoid nodules in the small intestine.

Physiological: The lymphatic system helps in tissue drainage, absorption of fats and fat-soluble substances from the intestinal villi of the small intestine and the process of immunity. The lymphatic organs take part in phagocytosis; white blood cells are produced and matured in lymphoid tissues, such as the red bone marrow, the thymus and the lymph nodes. The tonsils destroy inhaled or swallowed antigens.

The origin of a lymphatic capillary

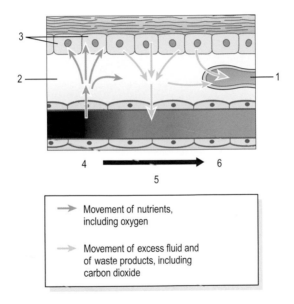

| Movement of nutrients, including oxygen |
| Movement of excess fluid and of waste products, including carbon dioxide |

Fig 34

1. Lymph capillary
2. Tissue fluid
3. Cells
4. Arterial end of the capillary
5. Flow of blood
6. Venous end of the capillary

Comments

Anatomical: The lymph capillaries have the same structure as the blood capillaries. However, they are more permeable, and they join to form lymph vessels along the arteries and veins. Muscular contraction, valves and arterial pulsatility facilitate the flow of lymph towards the thorax.

Physiological: Lymph is an interstitial fluid that is formed by the escape of plasma from the capillaries into the tissues, followed by diffusion across the permeable membrane of the lymph capillaries. It represents the amount of plasma that leaks out of the arterial capillaries, without going back into the venous capillaries. The lymph, drained by lymphatic vessels, carries plasma proteins, bacteria, organic waste products and lymphocytes. The plasma proteins go back into the bloodstream, and the cellular debris enters the lymph nodes, where it is filtered. The lymph carries nutrients towards the cells and removes their waste products.

Clinical: The amount of lymph in the body is about 3.5 L, and its composition resembles that of plasma. It looks like a clear watery fluid, except in the intestine, where it looks milky because of its fat content. The presence of oedema indicates a reduction in lymph drainage due to tissue compression, a surgical lesion or a structural anomaly in the lymph capillaries. The mechanics underlying the formation of lymph prevents the development of cardiovascular congestion, which can result from an overload of fluid, followed by an increase in blood volume.

Section through a lymphatic vessel, opened to show the cusps

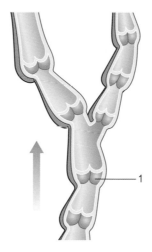

1

Fig 35

1. Semilunar cusp

Comments

Anatomical: Just like veins, the lymphatic vessels contain bicuspid valves that are made up of two cusps located all along their inner walls.

Physiological: The lymph is drained by lymphatic vessels with the help of valves that facilitate its flow towards the thorax and prevent reflux within the vessels. Muscular contraction and arterial pulsation help the lymphatic circulation.

Clinical: Lymphoedema of the lower leg that increases on standing, or is seen in chronic states, is a sign of a primary anomaly of the lymphatic system or secondary changes due to tissue compression, lymph node excision during cancer therapy or a parasitic infection, such as filariasis.

Section through a lymph node

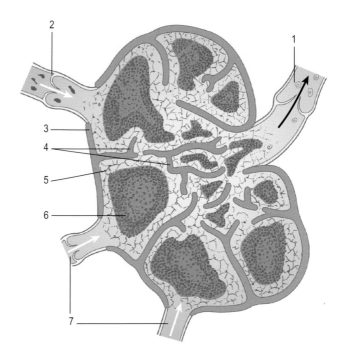

Fig 36 The *arrows* indicate the direction of lymph flow.

1. Efferent lymphatic vessel at the hilum of the node
2. Afferent lymphatic vessel
3. Capsule
4. Trabeculae
5. Reticular tissue
6. Primary follicle
7. Afferent lymphatic vessels

Comments

Anatomical: A lymph node is a bean-shaped organ of variable size that lies along the course of the lymphatic vessels. Its capsule is made up of fibrous tissues that penetrate the interior of the node to form the trabeculae. The substance of the node consists of reticular tissue that provides its framework and of lymphoid tissue that contains lymphocytes and macrophages. The capsule of the lymph node receives many afferent lymphatic vessels; its concave hilum admits one artery and gives off one vein and an efferent lymphatic vessel.

Physiological: The lymph flows successively through many lymph nodes that act as filters and sites of phagocytosis. They filter the lymph in the reticular and lymphoid tissues and destroy organic substances with the help of macrophages and antibodies. They also facilitate the proliferation of activated T- and B-lymphocytes, with the latter secreting antibodies that enter the lymph and the blood.

Clinical: Generally speaking, the lymph usually does not contain cellular waste products or foreign material when it re-enters the blood vascular system. A diseased lymph node is swollen and sometimes painful. It is a sign of activation of the immune system, whatever the location of the node (e.g., neck, groin, axilla), and of incomplete phagocytosis of an infectious agent or of a tumour.

Some lymph nodes of the face and neck

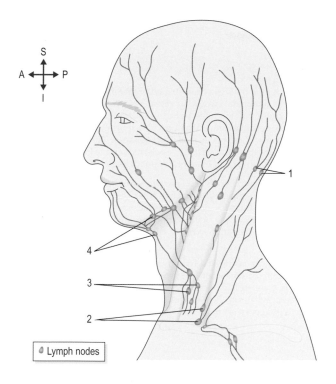

Lymph nodes

Fig 37

1. Occipital lymph nodes
2. Superficial cervical lymph nodes
3. Deep cervical lymph nodes
4. Submandibular lymph nodes

Comments

Anatomical: The lymph nodes exist in numerous superficial and deep groups that are distributed throughout the body.

Physiological: The deep and superficial lymph nodes drain the corresponding regions of the body. The cervical lymph nodes drain the lymph from the head and neck, the axillary lymph nodes from the upper limbs and the breasts, the mediastinal lymph nodes from the thoracic organs and tissues, the abdominal lymph nodes from the abdominal organs and tissues and the inguinal lymph nodes from the lower limbs.

Clinical: Examination of the lymph nodes entails searching for nodes to make a diagnosis and/or to establish the extent of spread in cases of infectious, inflammatory or neoplastic disease.

The spleen

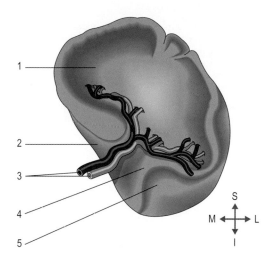

Fig 38

78

1. Gastric impression
2. Renal impression
3. Splenic artery and vein
4. Location of the tail of the pancreas
5. Colic impression

Comments

Anatomical: The spleen is an oval-shaped organ of variable size that lies in the left hypochondrium within the abdominal cavity. It has a very rich blood supply and is closely related to the stomach, the diaphragm, the left colic (splenic) flexure, the pancreas, the left kidney and the 9th, 10th and 11th ribs. It is made up of reticular tissue and lymphoid tissue. The splenic artery, which is a branch of the coeliac artery, and some nerve fibres enter the spleen, and the splenic vein and efferent lymphatic vessels leave it at the hilum.

Physiological: The spleen has the following functions: phagocytosis, immune defence and blood storage. It produces blood cells in the fetus and in the adult, when required. It stores about 350 mL of blood, which in cases of haemorrhage can be released into the circulation following stimulation from the sympathetic nervous system.

Clinical: The spleen is at high risk of haemorrhage because of its rich vascularity and its fragility. Abdominal trauma can lead to rupture; this is indicated clinically by pallor, sweating, tachycardia and assumption of the fetal position in order to reduce pain. The spleen can become enlarged in cases of cirrhosis, particularly in cases of lymphoma.

Section through the spleen

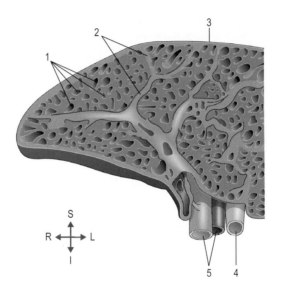

Fig 39

1. Splenic pulp
2. Trabeculae
3. Capsule
4. Lymphatic vessels
5. Splenic vein and splenic artery

Comments

Anatomical: The spleen is an oval-shaped abdominal organ, with a hilum on its inferior surface. Only its anterior surface is covered by peritoneum—its outer surface is covered by a fibroelastic capsule that extends inwards as trabeculae that enclose the splenic pulp, which consists of macrophages and lymphocytes. It consists of the red pulp and white pulp. The red pulp owes its colour to the red blood cells that are present in the large blood vessels. The white pulp, scattered throughout the red pulp, contains lymphocytes and macrophages. The hilum is the port of entry for the splenic artery and nerve fibres, and also the exit site for the splenic vein on its way to join the portal vein and for the efferent lymphatic vessel.

Physiological: The spleen produces blood cells in the fetus and, in the adult, when required. Its resident T- and B-lymphocytes are activated when presented with antigens. The spleen phagocytoses leukocytes, platelets and aged or abnormal red cells, releasing bilirubin and iron.

Clinical: In its normal state, the spleen is not palpable. When its volume is increased, as in splenomegaly, it becomes palpable and causes discomfort that is felt as a sense of heaviness in the left hypochondrium. Splenomegaly is a possible sign of a proliferation of lymphocytes, indicating an infection or a neoplastic process, such as a lymphoma.

The adult thymus and adjacent structures

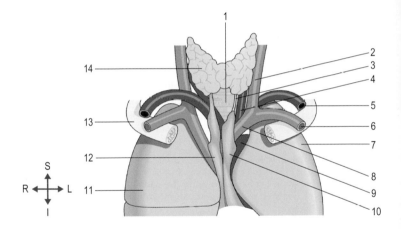

Fig 40

1. Trachea
2. Left internal jugular vein
3. Left recurrent laryngeal nerve
4. Left common carotid artery
5. Left subclavian artery
6. Left subclavian vein
7. Left lung
8. Left brachiocephalic vein
9. Aortic arch
10. Left lobe of thymus
11. Right lung
12. Right lobe of thymus
13. Right first rib
14. Thyroid gland

Comments

Anatomical: The thymus is an organ that is located in the superior mediastinum. Its relationships include the sternum, the heart and aortic arch, the lungs and trachea and the root of the neck. It consists of two lobes surrounded by a fibrous capsule and that is made up of a network of reticular cells and lymphocytes.

Physiological: The thymus plays a role in the in situ maturation of the stem cells of the lymphoid lineage. These are transformed into mature T-lymphocytes, which enter the circulation and the lymphatic tissues. These cells are able to react to a single antigen and to differentiate between the body's own cells and foreign cells.

Clinical: The thymus enlarges until puberty and then regresses and atrophies, which explains why, with age, T-lymphocytes react less efficiently with antigens. Coughing, dysphagia (difficulty in swallowing), a sense of heaviness or pain in the thorax and difficulty in breathing are all clinical signs of a thymoma.

Nervous system

The structure of neurones

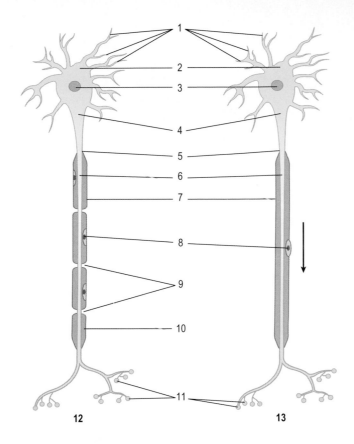

Fig 41 The *arrow* indicates the direction of conduction of the impulse.

1. Dendrites
2. Cell body
3. Nucleus
4. Axon hillock
5. Axolemma
6. Axon
7. Neurilemma
8. Nucleus of a Schwann cell
9. Nodes of Ranvier
10. Myelin sheath
11. Axon terminals
12. Myelinated nerve
13. Unmyelinated nerve

Comments

Anatomical: A nerve cell has a single axon whose membrane is called the *axolemma*. The axon and the dendrites, which are prolongations of the cytoplasm of the neurone, make up the white matter of the spinal cord. Outside the brain or the spinal cord, they are called *nerves* and make up the peripheral nervous system. The central nervous system consists of the brain and the spinal cord. Large axons or some of the peripheral nerves are covered by a myelin sheath produced by the Schwann cells. Myelin is a lipid rich substance. The neurilemma is the nerve sheath—the superficial layer of the plasma membrane of a Schwann cell—whereas the nodes of Ranvier correspond to the spaces between those cells.

Physiological: Neurones generate and transmit nervous or chemical impulses. The nodes of Ranvier allow the rapid transmission of nerve impulses in myelinated nerves.

Clinical: Sensory or motor loss is a sign of a reduction in the conduction of a nerve impulse. Local anaesthetics act by dampening painful thermal and tactile sensations. Inflammation in a tissue can give rise to pain on stimulation.

The arrangement of the myelin sheath

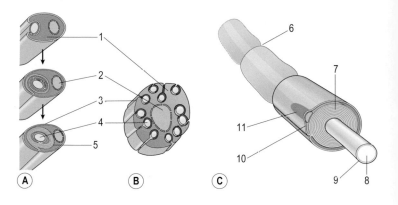

Fig 42 **(A)** Myelinated nerve. **(B)** Nonmyelinated nerve. **(C)** A length of a myelinated axon.

1. Cytoplasm of a Schwann cell
2. Nucleus of a Schwann cell
3. Neurilemma
4. Axon
5. Myelin sheath
6. Node of Ranvier
7. Myelin sheath
8. Axon
9. Axolemma
10. Neurilemma (sheath formed by the cytoplasm of Schwann cells)
11. Nucleus of a Schwann cell

Comments

Anatomical: A myelinated neurone has a large axon or peripheral nerves covered by a sheet of myelin, which is a lipid-rich substance. The neurilemma is the superficial layer of the plasma membrane of a Schwann cell, and the nodes of Ranvier correspond to gaps in the myelin sheath.

Physiological: The speed of nerve conduction increases with the diameter of the axon. It is greater in a myelinated nerve than in an unmyelinated nerve. In myelinated axons, the electrical events occur in the nodes of Ranvier.

Clinical: Sensory disturbances such as pins and needles, numbness and pain can affect various parts of the body (e.g., face, thorax, limbs). Changes in the conduction of the nerve impulse account for the clinical signs of the carpal syndrome and amyotrophic lateral sclerosis. The nerve impulse is also called the *action potential*. The rate of nerve conduction can be measured by electroneuromyography.

Diagram of a synapse: postsynaptic neurone

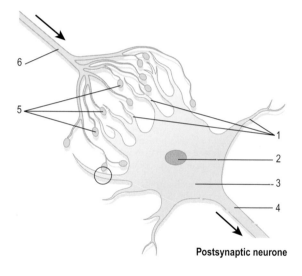

Postsynaptic neurone

Fig 43 The *arrow* indicates the direction of conduction of the impulse.

1. Dendrites
2. Nucleus
3. Cell body
4. Axon
5. Presynaptic terminals
6. Axon

Comments

Anatomical: The transmission of the nerve impulse requires multiple neurones that do not touch each other. The synapse is the functional zone between two neurones and is where the impulse is passed from the presynaptic neurone to the postsynaptic neurone. The axon of the presynaptic neurone terminates in presynaptic terminals that are full of synaptic vesicles.

Physiological: The synaptic vesicles contain a chemical substance known as the *neurotransmitter*, which is released into the synaptic cleft to reach its receptor on the membrane of the postsynaptic neurone.

Clinical: A neurotransmitter has many types of specific receptors. The presence or absence of certain receptors in the postsynaptic neurone is responsible for a specific chemical reaction that can excite or inhibit that neurone. There are at least 50 transmitters that stimulate or inhibit postsynaptic receptors, such as adrenaline, noradrenaline and dopamine.

Transverse section through a peripheral nerve, showing its protective coats

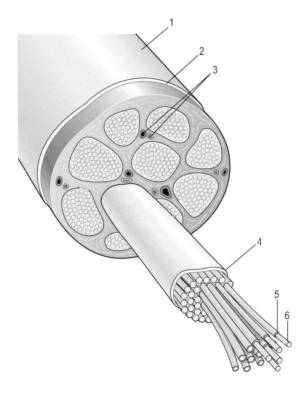

Fig 44

1. Nerve
2. Epineurium
3. Blood vessels
4. Perineurium
5. Endoneurium
6. Axon

Comments

Anatomical: Many neurones gather in bundles to form a nerve. Each bundle has many protective sheaths. The endoneurium and the perineurium are connective tissue sheaths that cover each fibre and each bundle of fibres, respectively; the epineurium is a connective tissue sheath covering multiple bundles of nerves.

Physiological: There are sensory, motor and mixed nerves. Sensory and motor nerves gather within the same connective tissue sheath to form a mixed nerve. The sensory nerves carry messages from the body to the spinal cord, and the motor nerves carry messages from the brain to the effector organs, which are skeletal muscles and smooth muscles for the motor nerves and the glands and heart for the autonomic nerves.

Clinical: The clinical signs of malfunction of nerves can vary in their expression and in their location. Such malfunction can cause paralysis, indicating a motor neurone lesion or pains, paraesthesia signifying a sensory neurone lesion or orthostatic hypotension, or erection–micturition disturbances, suggesting involvement of the autonomic nervous system. Intense pain can arise from a *peripheral neuropathy*, which is a general term referring to diseases of the peripheral nervous system.

Frontal section showing the meninges covering the brain and the spinal cord

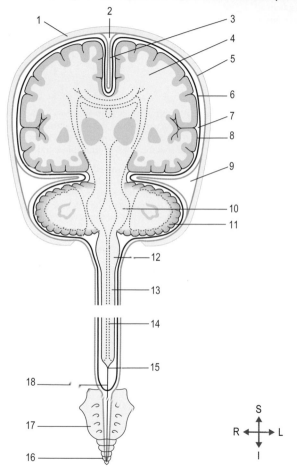

Fig 45

1. Cranial bone
2. Superior sagittal venous sinus
3. Falx cerebri
4. Cerebral hemisphere
5. The two layers of the dura mater
6. Arachnoid
7. Subarachnoid space
8. Pia mater adherent to the surface of the brain
9. Tentorium cerebelli and transverse venous sinus
10. Pons
11. Cerebellum
12. Medulla oblongata
13. Spinal cord
14. Central canal of the spinal cord
15. End of the spinal cord at the first lumbar vertebra
16. Coccyx
17. Sacrum
18. Filum terminale

Comments

Anatomical: The meninges include three tissue layers, which surround the brain and the spinal cord – the dura mater, the arachnoid mater and the pia mater. The space between the first two layers, called the *subdural space*, contains serous fluid; the space between the last two layers, called the *subarachnoid space*, contains the cerebrospinal fluid (CSF). The dura mater consists of two tissue layers covering the internal surface of the cranium and that of the brain. The space between these two layers is known as the *falx cerebri*. The arachnoid mater surrounds the spinal cord and fuses with the dura at the level of the second sacral vertebra. The pia mater contains the blood vessels and coats the cerebral convolutions and the spinal cord. It forms the filum terminale, which extends beyond the arachnoid and the dura on its way to fuse with the coccygeal periosteum.

Clinical: Headaches, vomiting, attention deficits and visual disturbances suggest intracranial hypertension – that is, an abnormal increase in intracranial pressure. The neurological signs, such as the state of consciousness, mydriasis and pupillary asymmetry, must be continuously evaluated. A score of 13/15 on the Glasgow scale is considered a criterion of severity, as are a rise in blood pressure, bradycardia and respiratory disturbances. Intracranial hypertension is due to an increase in volume of an intracranial component such as the brain, the blood vessels or the CSF. It can lead to cerebral oedema, coning or compression of the medulla oblongata, hypoxia or brain death.

The location of the cerebral ventricles: left lateral phantom view on the surface of the brain

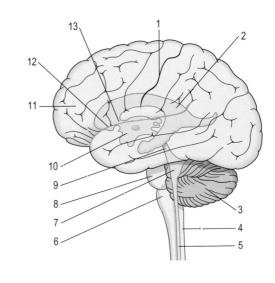

Fig 46

1. Central sulcus
2. Lateral ventricle
3. Cerebellum
4. Spinal cord
5. Central canal of the spinal cord
6. Medulla oblongata
7. Fourth ventricle
8. Pons
9. Cerebral aqueduct
10. Third ventricle
11. Cerebral hemisphere
12. Lateral sulcus
13. Interventricular foramen

Comments

Anatomical: The brain contains four ventricles—the right and left lateral ventricles, which are separated by the septum lucidum, and the third and fourth ventricles. The interventricular foramen is the site of communication with the third ventricle. The fourth ventricle, lying between the cerebellum and the pons, extends down to reach the central canal of the spinal cord.

Physiological: The CSF is secreted into all the ventricles by the choroid plexuses. It provides nutrition and protection for the brain and spinal cord. It maintains a constant level of humidity and pressure around these vital structures and acts as a shock absorber. Its circulation depends on the pulsations in the blood vessels, on breathing and on postural changes.

Clinical: Any significant increase in the size of the brain, due to a tumour or to a haemorrhage, reduces the amount of CSF, whereas any decrease in brain size due to degenerative changes or atrophy increases its amount. By reducing this pressure, a lumbar puncture can cause headaches or nausea. These signs need to be monitored after this procedure.

Frontal section of the cranium

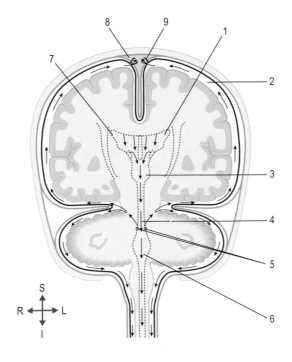

Fig 47 The *arrows* indicate the direction of flow of the cerebrospinal fluid.

1. Lateral ventricle
2. Subarachnoid space
3. Third ventricle
4. Cerebral aqueduct
5. Apertures in the roof of the fourth ventricle
6. Fourth ventricle
7. Lateral ventricle
8. Superior sagittal sinus
9. Arachnoid granulation

Comments

Physiological: The CSF, secreted into each of the four ventricles by the choroid plexuses, returns to the vascular system via the dural venous sinuses, into which the arachnoid granulations bulge; these act as unidirectional valves. A CSF pressure exceeding the venous pressure causes the CSF to flow into the blood, whereas the opposite causes the granulations to collapse, preventing the passage of blood constituents into the CSF.

Clinical: CSF contains water, mineral salts, glucose, plasma proteins and a few leukocytes, as well as small amounts of urea, creatinine, albumin and globulins.

Median section through the brain showing its main components

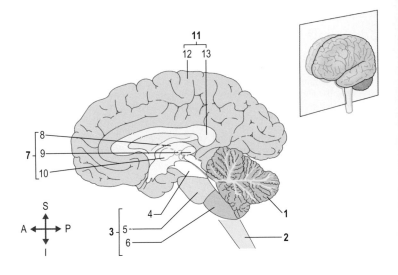

Fig 48

1. Cerebellum
2. Spinal cord
3. Brain stem
4. Mesencephalon
5. Pons
6. Medulla oblongata
7. Diencephalon
8. Thalamus
9. Pineal body
10. Hypothalamus
11. Cerebral hemisphere
12. Cerebral cortex
13. Corpus callosum

Comments

Anatomical: The brain, located in the cranial cavity, consists of the cerebral hemispheres, the diencephalon, the brain stem and cerebellum. Its arterial blood supply comes from the circle of Willis, and its venous blood drains into the dural venous sinuses.

Physiological: Intracranial blood flow is autoregulated by changes in the diameters of the arterioles, which adapt to variations in blood pressure to maintain a constant supply of glucose and oxygen to the brain. The purpose of this autoregulation is to ensure a constant blood flow to the brain to satisfy its needs for oxygen and nutrients.

Clinical: A fall in the supply of oxygen and nutrients to the brain causes neuronal dysfunction. If the oxygen deprivation is severe and lasts more than a few minutes, the brain will be irreversibly damaged.

The lobes and the main sulci of the cerebrum

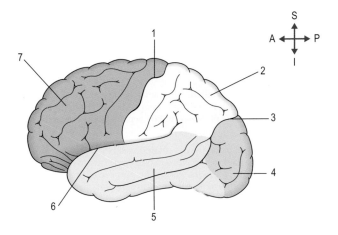

Fig 49 Left lateral view.

1. Central sulcus
2. Parietal lobe
3. Parieto-occipital sulcus
4. Occipital lobe
5. Temporal lobe
6. Lateral sulcus
7. Frontal lobe

Comments

Anatomical: The cerebral hemispheres lie inside the anterior and posterior cranial fossae. They are joined together by the corpus callosum, which is made up of white matter full of nerve fibres. The superficial layer of the hemispheres consists of grey matter made up of the cell bodies of the neurones, and its deep layer consists of nerve fibres, white matter and axons. The surface of the cerebral cortex contains sulci. Each hemisphere is divided into lobes, with each bearing the name of the corresponding cranial bone.

Clinical: Trauma to the head can cause damage to the scalp, the cranial bones, the meninges and the cerebrum. Such trauma is associated with vascular lesions, such as intracerebral haemorrhages. Scalp lesions are accompanied by a lot of bleeding but are mostly nonsevere. The most serious form of haemorrhage seen is an extradural haematoma, which can increase the intracranial pressure. It is due to an accumulation of blood between the cranial vault and dura mater and can be of venous origin (when the venous sinuses are damaged) or of arterial origin (e.g., when a meningeal artery is involved), and it can manifest itself many hours after the trauma. Haemorrhages can cause hypoxia and disturbances in cerebral blood flow.

Frontal section of the brain

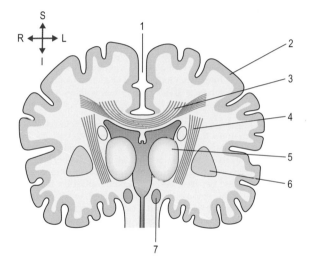

Fig 50 The important fibrous tracts are shown in *dark brown*.

1. Longitudinal cerebral fissure
2. Cerebral cortex
3. Corpus callosum
4. Internal capsule
5. Thalamus
6. Basal ganglia
7. Hypothalamus

Comments

Anatomical: The longitudinal cerebral fissure separates the right and left cerebral hemispheres, both of which contain a cerebral ventricle. These hemispheres are joined by white matter made up of nerve fibres, called the *corpus callosum*. The surface of the cerebral cortex bears sulci of variable depths. The internal capsule, carrying the motor fibres, lies between the midline nuclei (the basal ganglia) and the thalamus. These motor fibres, coursing inside the internal capsule, form the pyramidal or corticospinal tract and do not include the extrapyramidal motor fibres.

Physiological: The cerebral cortex is the seat of cognitive function (memory, reasoning and learning), sensory perception (sight, hearing, taste and smell), tactile and thermal perception, the feeling of pain and initiating voluntary movements.

Clinical: Clinical signs showing a decrease or loss of cognitive function in an individual suggest some form of damage to the cerebral cortex.

The left cerebral hemisphere and its main functional areas: left lateral view

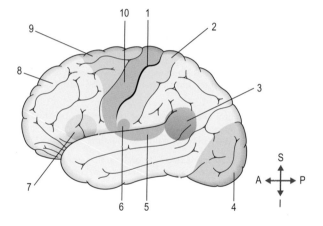

Fig 51

1. Central sulcus
2. Somatosensory area
3. Wernicke's speech area
4. Visual area
5. Auditory area
6. Gustatory area
7. Broca's motor speech area
8. Frontal area
9. Premotor area
10. Motor area

Comments

Anatomical: There are different functional areas in the brain—motor, sensory or associative. They are active in both hemispheres.

Physiological: The motor area controls the performance of voluntary movements, the sensory area controls sensory perception by receiving and decoding incoming neural messages, and the associative area integrates the cognitive functions, such as memorisation, reasoning, judgment, intelligence and the emotions.

Clinical: Any sign of impaired ability to move a part of the body suggests a lesion in the motor cortex. It can involve locomotion, the ability to grasp an object, the performance of a reflex, the ability to speak or write, mastication or deglutition and the ability to maintain an erect or sitting position. Similarly, any sign of sensory or associative deficiency indicates a lesion involving the corresponding functional area.

The pathways of the motor neurones: upper and lower motor neurones

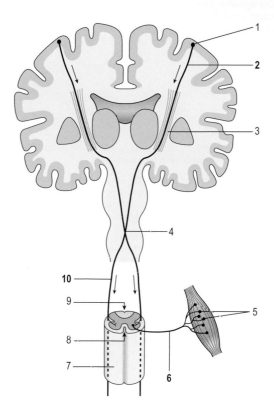

Fig 52

1. Cell body
2. Upper motor neurone
3. Internal capsule
4. Decussation of the pyramids in the brain stem
5. Motor end plate
6. Lower motor neurone
7. Spinal cord
8. Front
9. Back
10. Upper motor neurone

Comments

Anatomical: The precentral motor area lies in the frontal lobe, anterior to the central sulcus. Its cell bodies, pyramidal in shape, control the activity of the skeletal muscles.

Physiological: The upper and lower motor neurones participate in the spread of the nerve impulse. The upper neurone crosses the midline in the medulla oblongata and continues downwards on the opposite side of the body in the spinal cord. The term *decussation* is used to indicate this crossover. In the spinal cord, it synapses with a second motor neurone – the lower motor neurone – which then contacts its target muscle. Thus, the motor area of the right hemisphere controls voluntary movements on the left side of the body, whereas the left hemisphere controls those on the right side of the body.

Clinical: Any lesion in the left hemisphere causes clinical signs that are observable on the patient's right side and vice versa. For example, in cases of hemiplegia, a lesion in the left hemisphere causes paralysis on the right side of the body. Muscle weakness, along with spastic paralysis and muscle tremors, suggests an upper motor neurone lesion or pyramidal lesion. Muscular weakness, along with flaccid paralysis and muscular atrophy, suggests a lower motor neurone lesion.

Areas of the cerebral cortex involved in superior mental activities

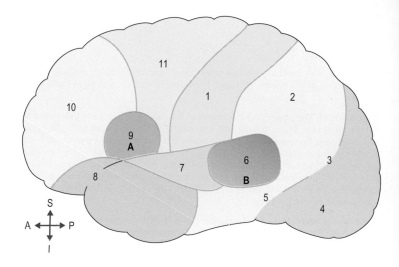

Fig 53

A. Motor area for speech.
B. Sensory area for speech.
1. Somatosensory
2. Spatial awareness of body and surroundings
3. Word visualization
4. Vision
5. Naming objects
6. Language, understanding and intelligence
7. Hearing
8. Behaviour, emotions and motivation
9. Phonation
10. Planning of complex movements and of thought
11. Motor

Comments

Anatomical: These areas are interconnected and are also connected to other cortical areas by means of association fibres.

Physiological: The association areas of the brain receive, coordinate and interpret inputs from the motor cortex and the sensory cortex to organise the cognitive functions. The premotor cortex in the frontal lobe coordinates movement; the prefrontal cortex mediates the perception of time, the ability to anticipate and control of the emotions. The sensory area in the temporal lobe deals with speech, understanding and intelligence. The part of the parieto-occipito-temporal area located in the parietal lobe is involved in space awareness, the interpretation of written language and the naming of objects.

Clinical: Any lesion involving one of these zones changes the various capabilities or functions of an individual.

The cerebellum and associated structures

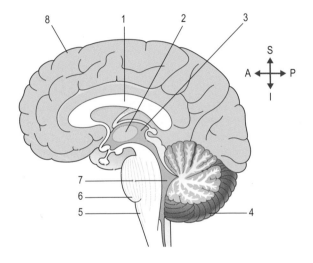

Fig 54

112

1. Corpus callosum
2. Thalamus
3. Third ventricle
4. Cerebellum
5. Medulla oblongata
6. Pons
7. Fourth ventricle
8. Cerebral cortex

Comments

Anatomical. The thalamus lies in the cerebral hemisphere just below the corpus callosum, on either side of the third ventricle. The hypothalamus lies below the thalamus, the cerebellum below the cerebral hemispheres and the midbrain below the cerebral hemispheres and above the pons, which separates the two hemispheres. The medulla oblongata lies adjacent to the pons.

Physiological: The cerebellum is involved in coordinating voluntary movements, posture and balance. The thalamus transmits signals to the cerebral cortex and plays a role in the perception of touch, pain, temperature and emotions. The hypothalamus forms part of the autonomic nervous system and controls appetite and satiety, thirst, water balance, emotions and the sleep cycle. The medulla oblongata contains part of the autonomic nervous system — the vital vasomotor and respiratory centres — and the midbrain mediates auditory and visual reflexes.

Clinical: Difficulty in coordinating voluntary movements and disturbances in balance associated with uncertain gait and movements suggest a cerebellar lesion.

The meninges covering the spinal cord

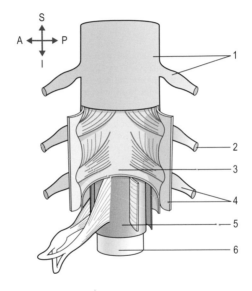

Fig 55 Some parts have been cut and removed to show the underlying layers.

1. Pia mater
2. Spinal nerve
3. Arachnoid mater
4. Dura mater
5. Pia mater
6. Spinal cord

Comments

Anatomical: The spinal cord forms part of the central nervous system. It is a neural tissue linking the brain to the rest of the body and has the shape of a cylinder encased inside the vertebral canal. It is surrounded by the meninges and bathed in CSF. It extends from the first cervical vertebra (the atlas) to the inferior border of the first lumbar vertebra. In adults, it measures about 45 cm. The meninges surround the spinal cord and consist of three tissue layers — the dura mater, the arachnoid mater and the pia mater. The dura mater, the outermost layer, is a rigid fibrous layer extending from the top of the cranial fossa to the upper part of the coccyx. It surrounds the brain, the spinal cord and the roots of the cranial and spinal nerves and the filum terminale. The arachnoid mater surrounds the brain, the cerebellum and the spinal cord, and lies between the dura mater and the pia mater.

Physiological: The nerve fibres descend into the spinal cord to transmit the signals from the brain to the organs and tissues. They leave the cord at different levels to reach their target structures. Conversely, the sensory nerves coming from the organs and tissues ascend in the spinal cord to reach the brain. The nerve impulses travel from synapse to synapse.

Clinical: Headaches, neck stiffness, fever, confusion, vomiting and photophobia (light intolerance) are signs of meningitis (inflammation of the meninges). A lumbar puncture performed to obtain a sample of CSF allows the diagnosis to be confirmed.

Transverse sections of the spinal canal showing the epidural space

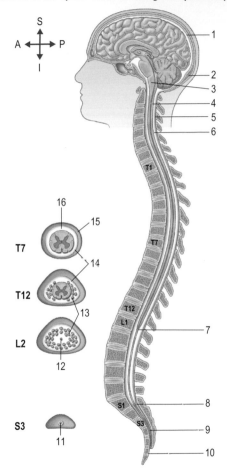

Fig 56

1. Dura mater
2. Occipital bone
3. Medulla oblongata
4. Spinal cord
5. Epidural space
6. Subarachnoid space
7. Lower extremity of the spinal cord
8. Lower extremity of the dural tube
9. Filum terminale
10. Coccyx
11. External filum terminale
12. Internal filum terminale
13. Nerve roots
14. Dura mater
15. Epidural space
16. Subarachnoid space

Comments

Anatomical: The dura mater, the arachnoid mater and the pia mater are the membranes that form the meninges. The dura is the rigid fibrous membrane extending from the top of the cranium to the upper part of the coccyx that surrounds the brain, the spinal cord, the roots of the cranial and spinal nerves and the filum terminale. The filum terminale is the fibrous extension of the pia mater. The epidural space lies between the dura and the tissues lining the vertebral canal. The subarachnoid space lies between the pia mater and the arachnoid mater.

Physiological: The spinal cord is functionally dependent on the brain and is independent only in cases in which spinal reflexes take over. The CSF flows from the ventricles towards the subarachnoid space.

Clinical: Peridural or epidural anaesthesia is initiated in the epidural space. An extradural haematoma is the accumulation of blood between the dura mater and an overlying cranial bone that can be lethal if the diagnosis is delayed.

The spinal cord and the spinal nerves

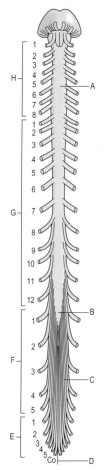

Fig 57

A. Spinal cord
B. Termination of the spinal cord
C. Cauda equina
D. Filum terminale
E. Sacral and coccygeal nerves
F. Lumbar nerves
G. Thoracic nerves
H. Cervical nerves
Co. Coccygeal plexus

Comments

Anatomical: The spinal cord is the neural tissue linking the brain to the rest of the body, with the exception of the cranial nerves. The filum terminale is the fibrous extension of the pia mater.

Physiological: The nerve fibres transmitting messages from the brain to the organs or from the organs to the brain leave or enter the spinal cord at the appropriate levels, which are named according to the segments involved — cervical, thoracic, lumbar, sacral and coccygeal nerves.

Clinical: Clinical signs localised at the level of the lower limbs and perineum, as well as problems with the sphincters, suggest the cauda equina syndrome. This is due to compression of the terminal region of the spinal cord distal to the conus medullaris; it involves nerves whose roots arise below the junction of L1 and L2 (the first two lumbar vertebrae) and are damaged at the levels of L2 to L5 and of the sacrococcygeal vertebrae, most frequently by the herniation of a disc. It needs to be treated urgently.

Transverse section of the spinal cord showing the nerve roots on one side

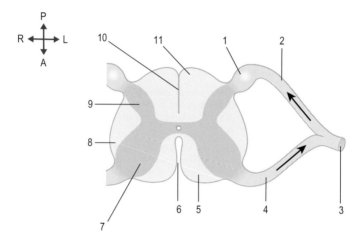

Fig 58

1. Dorsal root ganglion
2. Dorsal nerve root (sensory)
3. Mixed spinal nerve
4. Ventral nerve root (motor)
5. Anterior white column
6. Anterior median fissure
7. Anterior grey column
8. Lateral white column
9. Posterior grey column
10. Posterior median septum
11. Posterior white column

Comments

Anatomical: The spinal cord consists centrally of grey matter, which is surrounded by white matter. These structures are arranged in columns. The grey matter of the spinal cord is H-shaped, with two dorsal posterior horns, two ventral horns and two lateral horns. The cell bodies making up the spinal cord are composed of sensory neurons receiving messages from the periphery of the body, lower motor neurons transmitting signals to the muscles and interneurons linking the sensory and motor nerves. The dorsal root ganglion consists of the cell bodies of the sensory nerves. The white matter is made up of sensory and motor fibres, as well as the fibres of the interneurons.

Physiological: The impulses are transmitted from one neuron to another across the synapse. The cell bodies lying in the posterior columns of the grey matter are stimulated by sensory impulses coming from the body surface; their fibres, which make up the white matter, transmit these impulses to the brain. The cell bodies of the lower motor neurons, lying in the anterior columns of the grey matter, are stimulated by the axons of the upper motor neurons or by those of the interneurons. The cell bodies of these interneurons, belonging to the anterior and posterior columns, take part in the reflex arcs. The sensory or ascending nerves transmit the sensory impulses from the skin, the tendons, the muscles and the joints to the brain. The motor or descending nerves transmit the impulses from the cerebral cortex and cause the muscles to contract.

Clinical: Deficiency of vitamin B_{12}, which is needed for myelin synthesis, can cause degenerative changes in the spinal tracts.

One of the sensory pathways from the skin to the cerebral hemispheres

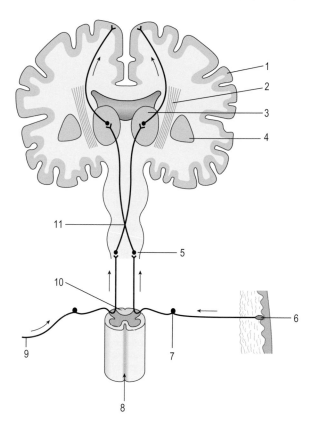

Fig 59

1. Cerebral cortex
2. Internal capsule
3. Thalamus
4. Basal ganglia
5. Cell bodies in the medulla oblongata
6. Sensory receptor in the skin
7. Dorsal root ganglion
8. Anterior aspect of the spinal cord
9. Peripheral spinal nerve
10. Dorsal white column
11. Medial lemniscal decussation

Comments

Anatomical: The white matter is arranged in columns made up of the fibres of sensory and motor neurons and those of interneurons.

Physiological: The skin, the tendons, the muscles and the joints have nerve endings that are sensory receptors. The impulses generated in these nerve endings are transmitted via three neurons before reaching the sensory area of the opposite cerebral hemisphere, where the message is interpreted and localised. The decussation, where the nerve fibres cross over to the opposite side of the body, is located in the medulla oblongata.

Clinical: The sensory receptors in the skin are stimulated by pain, cold, heat and pressure and give rise to painful thermal and tactile sensations.

The patellar (knee-jerk) reflex: left side

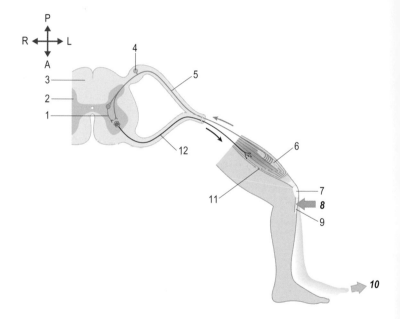

Fig 60

124

1. Interneuron (not involved in the stretch reflex)
2. Grey matter
3. Spinal cord
4. Dorsal root ganglion
5. Sensory neuron
6. Stretch receptor
7. Patella
8. Stimulus
9. Patellar tendon
10. Reaction
11. Quadriceps (effector muscle)
12. Motor neuron

Comment

Physiological: Two neurons take part in the knee-jerk reflex, which is a stretch reflex occurring when a tendon is stretched as it crosses a joint. Hitting the tendon below the flexed knee sets off a nerve impulse when the sensory nerve endings in the tendon and the muscles are stretched. The impulse reaches the cell body of the motor neuron located in the grey matter and causes the quadriceps femoris to contract and the foot to move forward.

Clinical: Reflexes occur rapidly. The feeling of pain in the brain and the motor response take place almost at the same time. This reflex guards against movements of the joint strong enough to damage the muscles, tendons and ligaments. The reflex is a test of the integrity of the reflex arc. It can be inhibited, particularly when nerve roots are compressed in cases of disc prolapse in the lumbar or cervical regions.

The relations between the sympathetic nervous system and the mixed spinal nerves

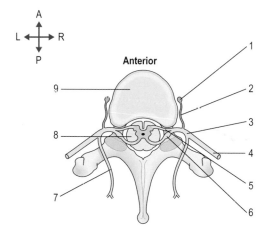

Fig 61 The sympathetic nervous system is in *green*.

1. Sympathetic ganglion
2. Grey ramus communicans
3. Mixed spinal nerve trunk
4. Ventral ramus (mixed)
5. Ventral root
6. Dorsal root ganglion
7. Posterior ramus (mixed)
8. Spinal cord
9. Body of a thoracic vertebra

Comments

Anatomical: The spinal nerves, arising from each side of the spinal cord, emerge from the intervertebral foramina as mixed nerves, formed by the fusion of a ventral motor root and a dorsal sensory root. The thoracic and lumbar spinal nerves receive preganglionic fibres from neurons of the autonomic nervous system. The ventral root consists of motor fibres, which are the axons of lower motor neurons located in the grey matter of the cord, and fibres of the sympathetic nervous system, which are the axons of cells located in the lateral column of the grey matter in the thoracic and lumbar regions. The dorsal nerve root is made up of sensory nerve fibres, and the dorsal root ganglion, lying at its exit from the spinal cord, consists of a group of cell bodies that send fibres to the peripheral sensory receptors and to the spinal cord.

Clinical: The sensory fibres supply a patch of skin, known as the *dermatome*. The location of sensory disturbances due to a dorsal root lesion allows one to define the level of nerve compression and pinpoint the location of the nerve damage precisely.

The meninges covering the spinal cord, the spinal nerves and their plexuses

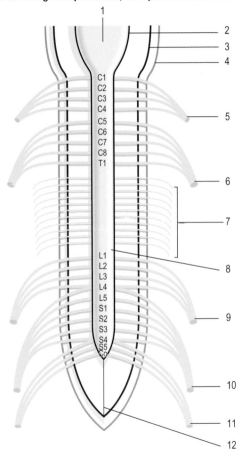

Fig 62

1. Brain stem
2. Pia mater
3. Arachnoid mater
4. Dura mater
5. Cervical plexus
6. Brachial plexus
7. Thoracic nerves 2 to 12 (nerves that do not belong to a plexus)
8. Spinal cord
9. Lumbar plexus
10. Sacral plexus
11. Coccygeal plexus
12. Filum terminale

Comments

Anatomical: The spinal nerves belong to the peripheral nervous system. There are 31 pairs of spinal nerves — 8 cervical, 12 thoracic, 5 lumbar, 5 sacral and 1 coccygeal. They are mixed nerves arising from each side of the spinal cord that exit through the intervertebral foramina. Each one is made up of a motor root and a sensory root. There are five plexuses of mixed nerves lying on either side of the vertebral column, located in the cervical, brachial, lumbar, sacral and coccygeal regions. These plexuses consist of collections of nerve fibres arranged so as to supply the skin, the bones, the muscles and the joints. There is no plexus in the thoracic region. The dura mater, the arachnoid mater and the pia mater are the three meningeal layers covering the brain and the spinal cord. The dura mater is the resistant external layer, the arachnoid mater is the intermediate layer and the pia mater is in contact with the brain and the spinal cord.

Physiological: Thus, tissues are innervated by multiple fibres from a plexus and not from a single spinal nerve. The arachnoid produces the CSF.

Clinical: A serious traumatic lesion of the brachial plexus caused, for example, by a motor vehicle accident, presents with signs and symptoms related to the entire arm and can even affect the diaphragm if the phrenic nerve is involved.

The cervical plexus, anterior view

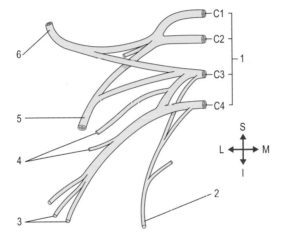

Fig 63

1. Nerve roots
2. Phrenic nerve for the diaphragm
3. Supraclavicular nerves
4. Nerve to the trapezius muscle
5. Transverse cervical nerve (cutaneous)
6. Great auricular nerve (for the side of the head)

Comments

Anatomical: The cervical plexus is formed by the ventral rami at the level of the first four cervical vertebrae (C1–C4). It lies deep to and is protected by the sternocleidomastoid muscle. The phrenic nerve, arising from the nerve roots of C3 to C5, descends into the thoracic cavity anterior to the pulmonary hilum.

Physiological: The cervical plexus supplies the head (its posterior and lateral aspects) and the neck (its anterior aspect down to the sternum, the sternocleidomastoid and the trapezius muscles). The phrenic nerve supplies the diaphragm and controls inspiration.

Clinical: A lesion or a trauma to the spinal cord at the level of the nerves of C3 to C5 can cause death by asphyxia, resulting from the cessation of spontaneous breathing secondary to damage to the phrenic nerve. Assisted ventilation becomes mandatory.

The main nerves of the upper limb

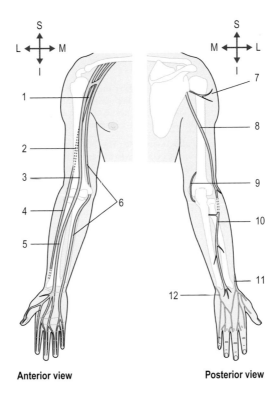

Anterior view

Posterior view

Fig 64

Anterior view

1. Radial nerve
2. Radial nerve behind the humerus
3. Median nerve
4. Radial nerve
5. Median nerve
6. Ulnar nerve

Posterior view

7. Axillary nerve
8. Radial nerve
9. Ulnar nerve
10. Branch of radial nerve
11. Radial nerve
12. Ulnar nerve

Comments

Anatomical: The brachial plexus is formed by the nerve roots of the last four cervical nerves and the first thoracic nerve. It lies partly in the axilla. It gives rise to the main nerves of the upper limb—the axillary, radial, median and ulnar nerves. They are mixed nerves containing sensory, motor and autonomic fibres.

Physiological: The axillary nerve supplies the deltoid muscle, the shoulder joint and the skin of the shoulder. The radial nerve supplies the triceps, the wrist extensors, the dorsum of the hand and the fingers (the thumb and the first three fingers). The median nerve supplies the muscles of the forearm, the hand and the fingers (the thumb and the second, third and fourth fingers). The ulnar nerve supplies the muscles of the forearm, the palm of the hand and the fourth and fifth fingers.

Clinical: Compression of the median nerve at the wrist (the carpal tunnel syndrome) can occur as the result of repeated movements of wrist flexion and extension or during pregnancy and gives rise to sensory symptoms and then to motor symptoms in all the fingers except the little finger, which is supplied by the ulnar nerve.

Distribution and origin of the cutaneous nerves of the upper limb

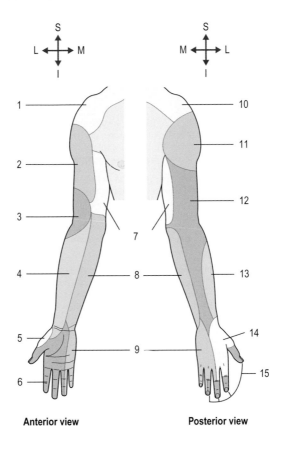

Anterior view

Posterior view

Fig 65 The various colours help distinguish the dermatomes.

Anterior view

1. Supraclavicular nerve (C3, C4)
2. Axillary nerve (C5, C6)
3. Radial nerve (C5, C6)
4. Musculocutaneous nerve (C5, C6)
5. Radial nerve (C7, C8)
6. Median nerve (C6–C8)
7. Medial cutaneous nerve of arm (C8, T1)
8. Medial cutaneous nerve of forearm (C8, T1)
9. Ulnar nerve (C8, T1)

Posterior view

10. Supraclavicular nerve (C3, C4)
11. Axillary nerve (C5, C6)
12. Radial nerve (C5, C6)
13. Musculocutaneous nerve (C5, C6)
14. Radial nerve (C7, C8)
15. Median nerve (C6–C8)

Comments

Anatomical: The cutaneous sensory nerves of the upper limb include the supraclavicular, the axillary, the radial, the musculocutaneous, the median and the ulnar nerves.

Physiological: The cutaneous nerves of the upper limb that arise at the level of the cervical vertebrae supply various parts of the upper limb. The dermatome corresponds to the skin area supplied by the same spinal nerve. The distribution of each nerve allows its area of supply to be visualised. The supraclavicular nerve supplies the base of the neck and the shoulder; the axillary nerve supplies the lateral aspect of the arm. The radial nerve supplies many areas, including the arm, the wrist, the hand and some fingers. The median and ulnar nerves supply the hand and some fingers; the musculocutaneous nerve supplies the forearm, and the medial cutaneous nerve supplies the medial border of the forearm.

Clinical: In cases of trauma to the upper limb, it is important to make an initial assessment of the extent of the damage to nerves with appropriate follow up. From knowledge of the sensory areas of the upper limb, one can identify the compressed nerve root in cases presenting with nerve pain involving the neck and the arm.

The lumbosacral and coccygeal plexuses

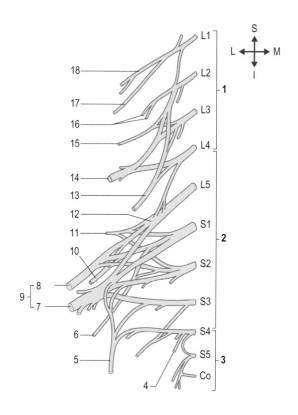

Fig 66

1. Lumbar plexus
2. Sacral plexus
3. Coccygeal plexus
4. Nerves supplying the levator ani, the coccygeus muscle and the external anal sphincter
5. Pudendal nerve
6. Posterior femoral cutaneous nerve
7. Tibial nerve
8. Common fibular nerve
9. Sciatic nerve
10. Inferior gluteal nerve
11. Superior gluteal nerve
12. Lumbosacral trunk
13. Obturator nerve
14. Femoral nerve
15. Lateral cutaneous femoral nerve
16. Genitofemoral nerve
17. Ilioinguinal nerve
18. Iliohypogastric nerve

Comments

Anatomical: The three lumbar sacral and coccygeal plexuses correspond to the numerous nerve fibres arising from the nerve roots in these regions. The lumbar plexus consists of fibres from the first four lumbar nerves, which lie anterior to the lumbar vertebrae and posterior to the psoas major. The sacral plexus, consisting of the ventral rami of the lumbosacral trunk and the first three sacral nerves, gives off the sciatic nerve, which contains fibres from L4 to S3, descends along the posterior part of the thigh and splits into the tibial nerve and common fibular nerve. The latter nerve divides into the superficial and deep fibular nerves. The coccygeal plexus is formed by the fibres of the fourth and fifth sacral nerves and the coccygeal nerve.

Physiological: The branches of the sciatic nerve supply the muscles in the posterior compartment of the thigh—the hamstring muscles. The tibial nerve and its branches supply the posterior part of the leg, the lateral aspect of the ankle, the heel, the sole of the foot, the dorsum of the foot and the toes. The femoral and obturator nerves supply the anterior aspect of the thigh. The iliohypogastric, ilioinguinal and genitofemoral nerves supply the inferior part of the abdomen, the upper part of the thigh and the inguinal region. The lateral femoral cutaneous nerve supplies the lateral, anterior and posterior aspects of the thigh. The common fibular nerve supplies the anterior aspect of the leg, the dorsum of the foot and the toes. The pudendal nerve supplies the external anal sphincter and the external urethral sphincter.

Clinical: Pain extending from the buttocks to the leg and the foot that follows the path of the sciatic nerve is typical of sciatica, commonly caused by a herniated disc. Intramuscular injections are administered in the superolateral quadrants of the buttocks to avoid any damage to the sciatic nerve.

The main nerves of the lower limb

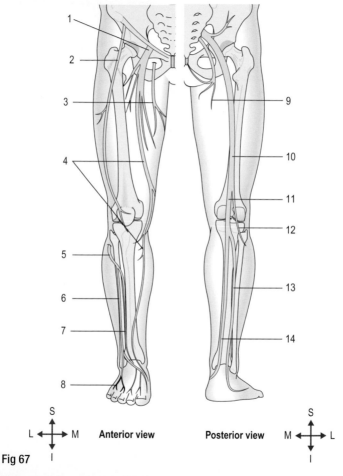

Fig 67

Anterior view

Posterior view

138

Anterior view

1. Femoral nerve
2. Lateral femoral cutaneous nerve
3. Obturator nerve
4. Saphenous nerve
5. Common fibular nerve
6. Superficial nerve
7. Deep fibular nerve
8. Sural nerve

Posterior view

9. Posterior femoral cutaneous nerve
10. Sciatic nerve
11. Tibial nerve
12. Common fibular nerve
13. Sural nerve
14. Tibial nerve

Comments

Anatomical: The main nerves of the lower limb belong to the lumbar plexus.

Physiological: The lateral femoral cutaneous nerve supplies the lateral, anterior and posterior aspects of the thigh. The femoral nerve supplies the anterior thigh muscles, and one of its branches, the saphenous nerve, supplies a part of the thigh, the ankle and the foot. The obturator nerve supplies the adductor muscles and the skin of the thigh. The sacral plexus supplies the muscles of the pelvic floor, the pelvic organs and the hip joint. The sciatic nerve supplies the hamstrings. The tibial nerve supplies the muscles and skin of the back of the leg and the plantar surfaces of the foot and toes. One of its branches, the sural nerve, supplies the heel, the ankle and the dorsum of the foot. The common fibular nerve supplies the muscles and skin of the front of the leg and the dorsal aspects of the foot and of the toes. The coccygeal plexus supplies the coccyx and the anus.

Clinical: Immobilisation, caused by a plaster cast or prolonged decubitus with the legs crossed, leads to compression of the common fibular nerve at the level of the fibular neck. This results in the steppage gait (foot drop with the foot hanging and the toes pointing down on walking) and also in a partial sensory loss in the anterolateral aspect of the thigh and anterior aspect of the instep.

Distribution and origin of the cutaneous nerves of the lower limb

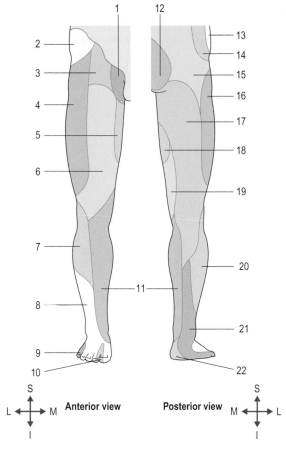

Fig 68 The various colours help distinguish the dermatomes.

Anterior view

1. Ilioinguinal nerve, L1
2. Subcostal nerve, T12
3. Genitofemoral nerve, L1, L2
4. Lateral femoral cutaneous nerve, L2, L3
5. Obturator nerve, L2–L4
6. Medial and intermediate femoral cutaneous nerves, L2, L3
7. Lateral sural cutaneous nerve, L5, S1, S2
8. Superficial fibular nerve, L4, L5, S1
9. Sural nerve, S1, S2
10. Deep fibular nerve, L4, L5
11. Saphenous nerve, L3, L4

Posterior view

12. Dorsal rami, S1–S3
13. Subcostal nerve, T12
14. Iliohypogastric nerve, L1
15. Dorsal rami, L1–L3
16. Lateral femoral cutaneous nerve, L2, L3
17. Posterior femoral cutaneous nerve, S1–S3
18. Obturator nerve, L2–L4
19. Medial femoral cutaneous nerve, L2, L3
20. Lateral sural cutaneous nerve, L4, L5, S1
21. Sural nerve, L5, S1, S2
22. Tibial nerve, S1, S2

Comments

Anatomical: The origins of the sensory cutaneous nerves of the lower limb are precisely located in the figure.

Physiological: The distribution of each nerve allows one to visualise the segment it supplies. The dermatome corresponds to the cutaneous area supplied by the same spinal nerve. Compression of the lateral femoral cutaneous nerve by tight clothing causes pain over a racquet-shaped area in the lateral aspect of the leg, known as *meralgia paraesthetica* or *lateral femoral cutaneous neuropathy*.

Cranial nerves and associated structures on the inferior aspect of the brain

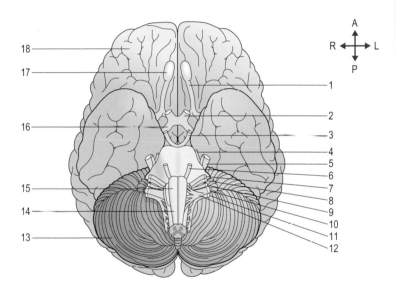

A
R ← → L
P

18
17
16
15
14
13

1
2
3
4
5
6
7
8
9
10
11
12

Fig 69

1. Olfactory nerve in the olfactory tract (I)
2. Optic nerve (II)
3. Oculomotor nerve (III)
4. Trochlear nerve (IV)
5. Trigeminal nerve (V)
6. Abducens nerve (VI)
7. Facial nerve (VII)
8. Auditory nerve (VIII)
9. Glossopharyngeal nerve (IX)
10. Vagus nerve (X)
11. Accessory nerve (XI)
12. Hypoglossal nerve (XII)
13. Cerebellum
14. Spinal cord
15. Medulla oblongata
16. Optic tract
17. Olfactory bulb
18. Cerebrum

Comments

Anatomical: There are 12 pairs of cranial nerves, numbered in Roman numerals according to the order of their sites of attachment to the brain. Their names indicate their functions and target areas. The sensory nerves are the olfactory, optic and auditory nerves. The motor nerves are the oculomotor, trochlear, abducens, accessory and hypoglossal nerves. The mixed nerves are the trigeminal, facial, glossopharyngeal and vagus nerves. The vagus nerve is also an important component of the parasympathetic nervous system.

Physiological: The olfactory nerve serves the sense of smell. The optic, ophthalmic, abducens, oculomotor, trochlear and a branch of the trigeminal all contribute to vision. The other branches of the trigeminal—the maxillary and the mandibular nerves—control mastication and also supply the face and the cranium. The facial nerve serves the sense of taste and supplies the muscles of facial expression. The vestibulocochlear nerve is the auditory nerve. The glossopharyngeal nerve contains sensory and motor fibres for the muscles of the tongue, the tonsils and the pharynx and takes part in swallowing and reflex vomiting. The vagus nerve supplies the smooth muscles and/or the secretory glands of the pharynx, larynx, trachea, bronchi, heart, oesophagus, stomach, intestine, exocrine pancreas, gall bladder and bile duct, spleen, kidneys and ureters and the blood vessels of the thoracic and abdominal cavities. The accessory nerve supplies the trapezius and sternocleidomastoid. By innervating the muscles of the tongue and those surrounding the hyoid bone, the hypoglossal nerve takes part in swallowing and phonation.

Clinical: Some fibres of the glossopharyngeal nerve carry nerve impulses from the carotid sinus and play a role in the control of arterial blood pressure.

Cutaneous distribution of the main branches of the right trigeminal nerve

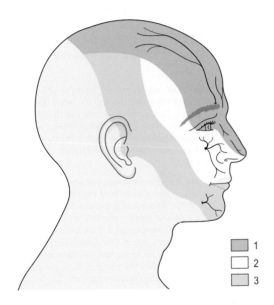

1
2
3

Fig 70

1. Ophthalmic nerve
2. Maxillary nerve
3. Mandibular nerve

Comments

Anatomical: The trigeminal nerve is a large mixed cranial nerve containing both sensory and motor fibres. It has three main branches—the ophthalmic, maxillary and mandibular nerves.

Physiological: The trigeminal nerve is the main sensory nerve of the face and of the cranium. Its sensory fibres carry impulses from the pain, temperature and touch receptors in the nasal and buccal cavities and in the teeth. Its motor fibres stimulate the muscles of mastication. The ophthalmic nerve, a sensory nerve, supplies the nasal mucosa, the lacrimal gland, the conjunctiva and the eyelid, the forehead and the scalp. The maxillary nerve, also a sensory nerve, supplies the cheek, the upper gums and teeth and the lower eyelid. The mandibular nerve, a mixed nerve, is both motor and sensory and supplies the lower teeth and gums, the external acoustic meatus and the tympanum, the lower lip, the chin, the mandible and the tongue. Its motor fibres participate in mastication.

Clinical: The occurrence of acute, paroxysmal, recurring and disabling pains in the face suggest a lesion of the trigeminal nerve, a trigeminal neuralgia.

Location of the vagus nerve in the thorax, seen from the right side of the body

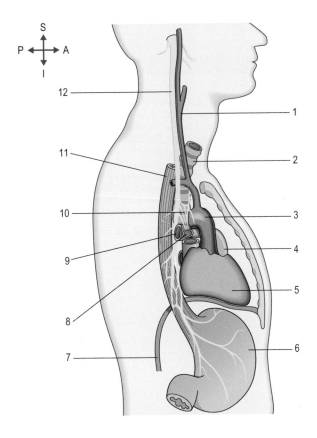

Fig 71

1. Common carotid artery
2. Trachea
3. Aortic arch
4. Pulmonary trunk
5. Heart
6. Stomach
7. Diaphragm
8. Right pulmonary artery
9. Right bronchus
10. Cardiac plexus
11. Oesophagus
12. Vagus nerve

Comments

Anatomical: The vagus nerve is the 10th cranial nerve. It is mixed, containing both sensory and motor fibres, which run along the neck and through the thorax and the abdomen. It contains parasympathetic fibres and is an important component of the parasympathetic nervous system.

Physiological: The vagus supplies motor and sensory fibres to the oropharyngolaryngeal region, the soft palate, the pharynx and the larynx and controls the vegetative activities of the cardiorespiratory organs (the heart, the thoracic and abdominal blood vessels, the lungs, the trachea and the bronchi), the alimentary system (the oesophagus, the stomach, the intestine, the exocrine pancreas, the gall bladder and the bile ducts), the spleen and the kidneys and ureters.

Clinical: Stimulation of the vagus results in constriction of the bronchi, increased production of saliva and digestive juices and activation of the smooth muscle of the alimentary tract.

The sympathetic nervous system: its main targets and its stimulatory effects

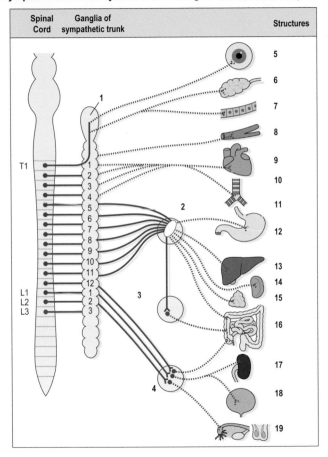

Fig 72

1. Superior cervical ganglion
2. Coeliac ganglion
3. Superior mesenteric ganglion
4. Inferior mesenteric ganglion
5. Dilator pupillae muscle
6. Salivary glands
7. Buccal and nasal mucosae
8. Skeletal blood vessels
9. Heart
10. Coronary arteries
11. Trachea and bronchi
12. Stomach
13. Liver
14. Spleen
15. Suprarenal medulla
16. Colon and small intestine
17. Kidney
18. Bladder
19. Sex organs and external genitalia

Comments

Anatomical: Pre- and postganglionic neurones take part in the transmission of nerve impulses of the sympathetic system. The preganglionic neurones lie in the thoracic and lumbar segments of the spinal cord. Their cell bodies are located in the grey matter, and their nerve fibres leave the spinal cord via the anterior root to reach a prevertebral ganglion. The postganglionic neurones have their cell bodies in a ganglion and, from there, they send their fibres to the target organ or tissue. Chains of sympathetic ganglia extend from the neck to the sacrum on either side of the vertebral bodies. As they leave the spinal cord, the fibres of the preganglionic neurones synapse with the cell bodies of the nearby postganglionic neurones.

Physiological: Stimulation of the sympathetic nervous system produces dilation of the pupils, vasodilation in the coronary arterial system, bronchodilation, relaxation of the smooth muscle of the bladder, ejaculation in men, inhibition of mucus secretion of salivary glands in the buccal and nasal mucosae and urine formation in the kidney; reduced gastric and intestinal peristalsis; contraction of the heart, the spleen and the sphincters of the colon, the small intestine and the bladder; enhancement of blood coagulation, hepatic glycogenesis and glandular secretion in the sex organs. Thus, it allows the body to face situations of excitement, nervous tension or emotional upset.

The parasympathetic nervous system: its main targets and its stimulatory effects

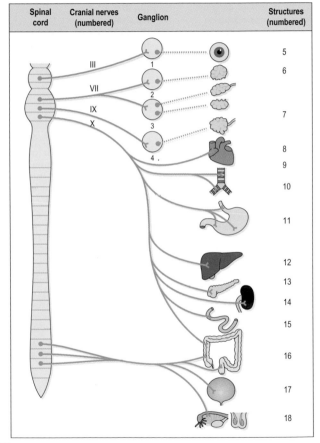

Fig 73

1. Ciliary ganglion
2. Pterygopalatine ganglion
3. Submandibular ganglion
4. Optic ganglion
5. Iris
6. Lacrimal gland
7. Salivary glands—submandibular, sublingual and parotid
8. Heart
9. Coronary arteries
10. Trachea and bronchi
11. Stomach
12. Liver and gall bladder
13. Pancreas
14. Kidney
15. Small intestine
16. Large intestine
17. Bladder
18. Sex organs and external genitalia

Comments

Anatomical: Two neurones are needed to transmit the nerve impulse to the affected organ. Acetylcholine is the neurotransmitter released by preganglionic fibres in the sympathetic ganglia; noradrenaline is the neurotransmitter released in the effector organs of the sympathetic nervous system.

Physiological: Stimulation of the parasympathetic nervous system causes contraction of the pupils, the trachea and bronchi and the bladder wall; erection; relaxation of the vesical and intestinal sphincters; a drop in the frequency and force of the heartbeat; enhanced secretion of tears, saliva, gastric and pancreatic juices, bile and urine; enhanced digestion and gastric and intestinal peristalsis. The overall effect of its activation is to allow digestion and restorative processes in the body to take place in peace and quiet.

Clinical: Vasovagal syncope, associated with bradycardia and hypotension, with possible loss of consciousness, is due to overactivity of the parasympathetic nervous system in certain circumstances, such as prolonged standing, exposure to confined spaces, severe pain and the sight of blood.

Sense organs

The components of the ear

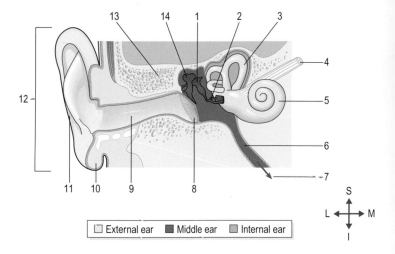

Fig 74

1. Incus
2. Stapes
3. Semicircular canal
4. Vestibulocochlear nerve
5. Cochlea
6. Auditory (pharyngotympanic or eustachian) tube
7. Towards the nasopharynx
8. Tympanic membrane
9. External acoustic meatus
10. Lobule
11. Helix
12. Auricle
13. Temporal bone
14. Malleus

Comments

Anatomical: The ear is made up of three separate parts — the external ear, the middle ear and the internal ear. The external ear consists of the auricle and the external acoustic meatus, made up of fibrocartilage and osteocartilage, respectively. The middle ear consists of the tympanic membrane, which separates the external acoustic meatus from the tympanic cavity, the three ossicles, the malleus (or hammer), the incus (or anvil) and the stapes (or stirrup); the mastoid bone and the eustachian tube, which connects the tympanic cavity to the nasopharynx. The internal ear is made up of the bony and the membranous labyrinths, consisting of the cochlea and the vestibule.

Physiological: The ear is the auditory organ responding to sound, which is due to air vibration. The external ear picks up the sound waves and transmits them to the middle ear as they are amplified by the vibrations of the tympanic membrane. The middle ear then transmits the sound vibrations towards the internal ear, mobilising the auditory ossicles, the perilymph and the endolymph. The internal ear then transmits a fluid pressure wave to the organ of Corti. The neurosensory cells transform this mechanical signal into an electrical signal, which is conveyed by the vestibulocochlear nerve (the cranial nerve VIII) to the brain stem.

Clinical: The clinical signs and symptoms of dysfunction of the ear include pain, ringing in the ear, partial or total (unilateral or bilateral, acute or chronic) hearing loss, otorrhoea (leakage of blood, pus or cerebrospinal fluid) and vertigo.

The auditory ossicles

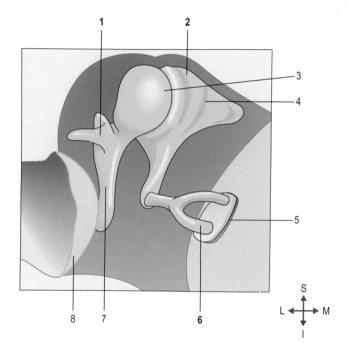

Fig 75

156

1. Malleus (hammer)
2. Incus (anvil)
3. Head
4. Body
5. Oval window of the vestibule
6. Stapes (stirrup)
7. Handle of the malleus
8. Tympanic membrane

Comments

Anatomical: The three ossicles—the malleus (hammer), incus (anvil) and stapes (stirrup)—are the auditory ossicles of the middle ear. Held in place by their ligaments, they are linked by joints and operate as a unit. The handle of the malleus is in contact with the tympanic membrane, and its head is linked to the incus (the intermediate ossicle). The incus is linked to the stapes (the third ossicle), which is attached to the oval window of the vestibule.

Physiological: The vibrations of the membrane are transmitted to the three ossicles. The movements of the stapes (the third ossicle) generate across the oval window of the vestibule fluid waves in the perilymph of the scala vestibuli, which are transmitted to the cochlear duct.

Clinical: The auditory threshold is at 0 decibels (dB), and the pain threshold is at 130 dB. Injury to the external or middle ear causes conductive deafness. Signs and symptoms of acute otitis media include fever, earache, partial hearing loss, sometimes with purulent discharge.

The internal ear: the membranous labyrinth inside the bony labyrinth

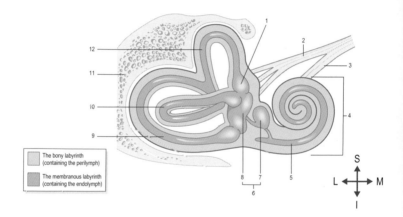

The bony labyrinth
(containing the perilymph)

The membranous labyrinth
(containing the endolymph)

Fig 76

1. Ampulla of the anterior semicircular canal
2. Vestibular nerve
3. Cochlear nerve
4. Cochlea
5. Cochlear duct
6. Vestibule
7. Saccule
8. Utricle
9. Posterior semicircular canal (membranous)
10. Lateral semicircular canal (membranous)
11. Temporal bone
12. Anterior semicircular canal (membranous)

Comments

Anatomical: The internal ear consists of two parts, the bony labyrinth and the membranous labyrinth, and three regions – the vestibule containing the utricle and the saccule, the semicircular canals lying in the three planes of space, and the cochlea. The bony labyrinth contains the membranous labyrinth, which floats in the perilymph and is filled with endolymph. The vestibule contains two membranous sacs, the utricle and the saccule. The cochlear duct is the part of the membranous labyrinth at which the ciliated cochlear cells give rise to the auditory receptors in the organ of Corti.

Physiological: The internal ear is the organ responsible for hearing and balance. By transforming fluid waves into electrical signals, the internal ear plays in a role in hearing. The utricle and the saccule, which form part of the vestibule, along with the semicircular canals, are responsible for the maintenance of balance.

Clinical: A lesion of the internal ear can cause sensorineural deafness and balance problems. An isolated and brief attack of vertigo, caused by the circular movement of the head, is typical of benign paroxysmal positional vertigo. A more severe attack of vertigo of longer duration is suggestive of Ménière's disease or of vestibular neuritis.

Transverse section of the cochlea showing the spiral organ (of Corti)

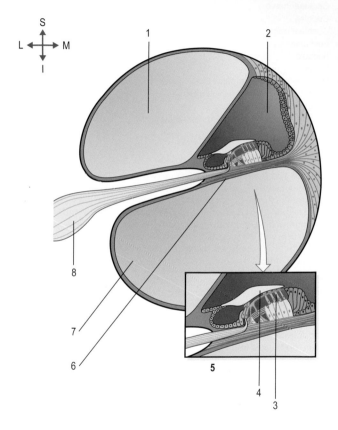

Fig 77

1. Scala vestibuli (perilymph)
2. Cochlear duct (endolymph)
3. Hair cell
4. Tectorial membrane
5. Spiral organ
6. Basilar membrane
7. Scala tympani (perilymph)
8. Vestibulocochlear nerve, cochlear part

Comments

Anatomical: The cochlea, shaped like the shell of a snail, is made up of the scala vestibuli, the cochlear duct and the scala tympani. The cochlear duct contains the hair cells carrying the auditory receptors, which make up the spiral organ of Corti. The scala tympani and the scala vestibuli contain a fluid known as perilymph, whereas the cochlear duct contains endolymph. The auditory receptors are the dendrites of the sensory nerves that cluster to form the cochlear part of the vestibulocochlear nerve.

Physiological: Vibrations in the organ of Corti cause deformation of the stereocilia of the neurosensory cells, inducing a depolarising action potential, which will be transmitted by the vestibulocochlear nerve (the combined cranial nerve VIII) to the brain. The vestibulocochlear nerve has two functions, hearing and balance.

Clinical: A change in the position of the head provokes a movement in the perilymph and endolymph, which will set in motion the stereocilia of the hair cells and stimulate the sensory receptors. Balance is maintained by an antagonism between the two ears, with an increase in the vestibular activity in one ear and a decrease in the other ear.

The transmission of sound waves

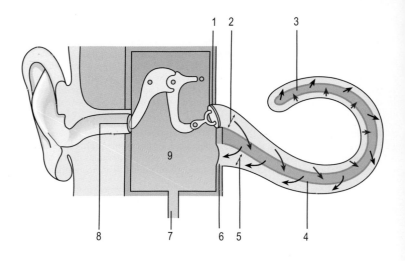

Fig 78 The ear is shown with the cochlea unwound.

1. Oval window of vestibule
2. Scala vestibuli
3. Cochlear duct
4. Basilar membrane and spiral organ of Corti
5. Scala tympani
6. Round window of cochlea
7. Auditory (eustachian) tube
8. Tympanic membrane
9. Chain of auditory ossicles

Comments

Physiological: In the external ear, the auricle picks up the sound waves from the air and transmits them to the middle ear by causing the tympanic membrane to produce vibrations and amplify them. The middle ear then transmits these vibrations to the inner ear via the mechanical motion of the ossicles. The motion of the last ossicle (the stapes), acting across the oval window, generates fluid waves in the perilymph of the scala vestibuli, which are reflected towards the cochlear duct. The waves produced in the endolymph then cause the basilar membrane to vibrate and stimulate the receptors of the hair cells of the spiral organ. Sounds of different frequencies stimulate the basilar membrane at different points. The nerve impulses thus produced are then transmitted to the brain via the auditory portion of the vestibulocochlear nerve.

Clinical: The amplitude of a sound wave is measured by its frequency in hertz (Hz). Its intensity depends on the amplitude of the stimulus that sets it off. Exposure to a loud noise can damage the hair cells of the spiral organ of Corti and cause deafness, especially if it is of long duration.

Cross section of the eye

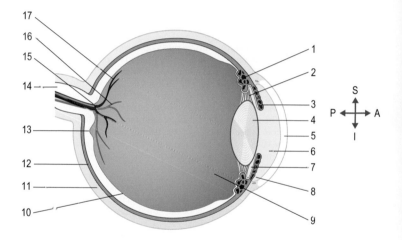

Fig 79

1. Ciliary body
2. Suspensory ligament of lens
3. Iris
4. Lens
5. Cornea
6. Anterior chamber
7. Posterior chamber
8. Scleral venous sinus (canal of Schlemm)
9. Vitreous body
10. Retina
11. Sclera
12. Choroid
13. Macula
14. Optic nerve
15. Optic disc
16. Retinal vein
17. Retinal artery

Comments

Anatomical: The eye lies in the orbital cavity and is made up of an outer coat, internal structures and adnexal structures. The outer coat consists of three layers—a fibrous external layer composed of the sclera (the white of the eye), which is continuous with the cornea, an intermediate vascular layer containing the choroid (the vascular layer of the eye), and continuous with the ciliary body and the iris, and an inner nervous layer made up of the retina, which lies between the choroid and the vitreous body. The internal structure of the eye consists of the lens, the aqueous humour and the vitreous body. The adnexal structures of the eye comprise the eyelids, the conjunctiva, the lacrimal glands, the lacrimal ducts and the oculomotor muscles. The eye is supplied by the ciliary arteries and the central retinal artery and vein, and it is innervated by the optic nerve.

Physiological: The eye is the visual organ. Although separate, the two eyes function as a pair, with coordinated actions. The sclera gives the eye its shape and provides sites of attachment for the ocular muscles. The rays of light penetrate the eye at the level of the pupil and are refracted by the cornea, which allows them to reach the retina. The role of the retina is to transform light energy into electrical energy, which is then transmitted to the brain via the optic nerve.

Clinical: Monocular vision—using one eye—is possible but is associated with a reduced ability to judge distances in space and see the world properly in three dimensions.

The choroid, the ciliary body and the iris (frontal view)

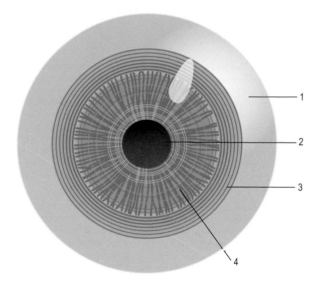

Fig 80

1. Choroid
2. Pupil
3. Ciliary body
4. Iris, with circular and meridional fibres of the ciliary muscle

Comments

Anatomical: The choroid lines most of the internal surface of the sclera. It is richly vascular and dark in colour and is continuous with the ciliary body, which is made up of the ciliary muscle fibres and is supplied by the parasympathetic fibres of the oculomotor nerve (III). The iris is a coloured ring containing the pigmented cells in the anterior part of the eye; it divides the eye into the anterior and posterior chambers, both of which contain the aqueous humour. It consists of two layers of smooth muscle and encloses the centrally located pupil. The iris is supplied by sympathetic and parasympathetic fibres.

Physiological: The choroid absorbs light after it passes through the retina. The ciliary body secretes the aqueous humour, and its muscle fibres control the size and thickness of the lens. Stimulation of the oculomotor nerve causes the ciliary muscle to contract and produce accommodation. On stimulation, the parasympathetic nerve fibres cause contraction of the pupil, whereas the sympathetic nerve fibres cause dilation.

Clinical: The colour of the iris is a genetic trait and depends on the number of pigmented cells present. Persons with blue eyes have a smaller number of pigmented cells than those with brown eyes. People with albinism have no pigmented cells at all.

The lens and its suspensory ligament: frontal view

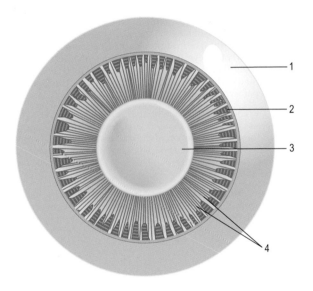

Fig 81 The iris has been removed.

1. Sclera
2. Ciliary body
3. Lens
4. Suspensory ligaments

Comments

Anatomical: The lens is a circular biconvex elastic structure located behind the pupil; its thickness is controlled by the ciliary muscles, to which it is attached by its suspensory ligaments.

Physiological: The lens refracts the light rays. Its ability to refract varies according to its thickness, which is controlled by the contraction of the ciliary muscles acting on its suspensory ligaments. The lens allows the eye to focus and form an image of an object on the retina.

Clinical: The closer the object, the greater the contraction of the ciliary muscles as they increase the thickness of the lens and allow focusing to take place with the formation of an image of an object on the retina.

Magnified section of the retina

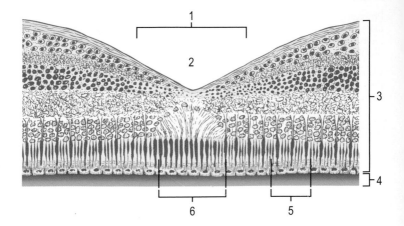

Fig 82

1. Macula
2. Fovea centralis
3. Retina
4. Choroid
5. Rods and cones
6. Cones only

Comments

Anatomical: The retina, the deep layer of the wall of the eye, lies between the choroid and the vitreous body. It consists of multiple layers of nerve cell bodies and their axons, as well as layers of pigmented epithelial cells. The light-sensitive layer consists of rods and cones, which contain photosensitive pigments and are the sensory receptors able to transform light into nerve impulses. The fovea centralis is the central part of the macula lutea (the yellowish area) and contains only cones.

Physiological: The sensory receptor cells, the rods and the cones, are responsible for transforming light into nerve impulses.

Clinical: Visual acuity is maximal at the fovea centralis. In the developed world, senile macular degeneration is the first cause of loss of vision in people older than 60 years and is due to progressive destruction of the macula.

The optic nerves and their pathways

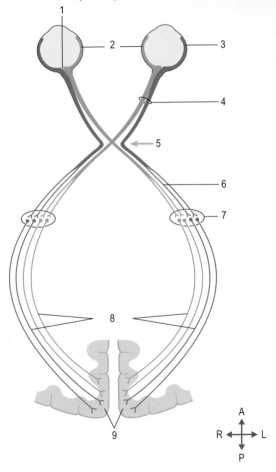

Fig 83

1. Macula
2. Nasal retina
3. Temporal retina
4. Optic nerve
5. Optic chiasma
6. Optic tract
7. Lateral geniculate body
8. Optic radiations
9. Visual area in the occipital lobe of the cerebrum

Comments

Anatomical: As they leave the retina, the fibres of the optic nerve converge to form the optic nerve near the nasal border of the macula. This nerve, cranial nerve II, crosses the choroid, the sclera, the orbital cavity and the optic foramen of the sphenoid bone before joining its mate from the contralateral eye to form the optic chiasma.

Physiological: At the chiasma, fibres from the nasal side of each retina cross the midline and change sides, whereas the fibres from the temporal side do not cross the midline. Thus, each optic tract after the chiasma contains fibres coming from the nasal and temporal sides of the retina. These fibres synapse with cell bodies of the lateral geniculate body in the thalamus and then proceed, as optic radiations, to reach the visual area in the occipital lobe of the cerebrum.

Clinical: Partial or complete loss of visual acuity or pain suggests an optic neuritis or some damage to the optic nerve.

Section of the eye showing the focusing of light rays on the retina

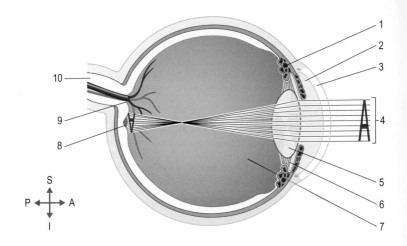

Fig 84

1. Ciliary muscle
2. Aqueous humour
3. Cornea
4. Light rays entering the eye
5. Lens
6. Suspensory ligament of lens
7. Vitreous body
8. Macula
9. Optic disc
10. Optic nerve

Comments

Anatomical: As they enter the eye, light rays cross many areas with fixed refractory indices, such as the conjunctiva, the cornea, the aqueous humour and the vitreous body, and also the lens, with its variable refractory index.

Physiological: The biconvex lens refracts and focuses the light rays. The image formed in the retina is inverted; it is turned the right way up by the brain.

Clinical: As the object gets nearer, refraction must increase. Disorders of refraction (myopia and farsightedness) are corrected using biconvex or biconcave lenses as contact lenses or eyeglasses.

Accommodation: how the ciliary muscle alters the shape of the lens

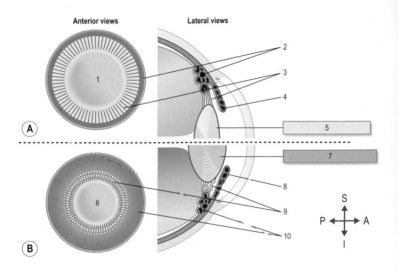

Anterior views   Lateral views

1

2

3

4

5

6

7

8

9

10

S

P ←→ A

I

A

B

Fig 85 (A) Accommodation of the eye for distance vision. The ciliary muscle relaxes, the suspensory ligaments are tightened and the lens is flattened.
(B) Accommodation of the eye for near vision. The ciliary muscle contracts, the suspensory ligaments relax and the lens becomes more convex.

1. Lens
2. Relaxed ciliary body
3. Contracted suspensory ligaments
4. Iris
5. Lens for distant vision
6. Lens
7. Lens for near vision
8. Iris
0. Relaxed suspensory ligaments
10. Contracted ciliary muscle

Comments

Physiological: By changing its size, the pupil controls the amount of light entering the eye. Stimulation of the oculomotor nerve causes the ciliary muscle to contract, allowing accommodation to occur. Stimulation of the parasympathetic nerves causes contraction of the pupil, whereas stimulation of the sympathetic fibres causes dilation of the pupil. Accommodation, which is needed to look at nearby objects, occurs as a result of pupillary constriction, which reduces the width of the light beam entering the eye and focuses it on the convex central part of the lens. The ocular muscles mobilise the eyes, enhancing their convergence towards the object being looked at. The closer the object, the greater the degree of convergence required. Changes in lens thickness allow light to be focused on the retina, depending on the refractive index of the lens. A bright light makes the pupils contract, whereas a dim light makes them dilate. During accommodation for near vision, the ciliary muscle contracts, the suspensory ligaments relax and the lens becomes more convex. During accommodation for distant vision, the ciliary muscle relaxes, the suspensory ligaments become taut and the lens becomes flatter.

Clinical: Clear vision depends on the size of the pupils and on the stimulation of the corresponding areas in both retinas. Night vision is weak because the cones are not strongly stimulated. Diplopia (double vision) is due to incomplete convergence on the object. Long-sightedness is related to ageing of the lens, which loses its elasticity and becomes more rigid.

The components of the visual field: monocular and binocular vision

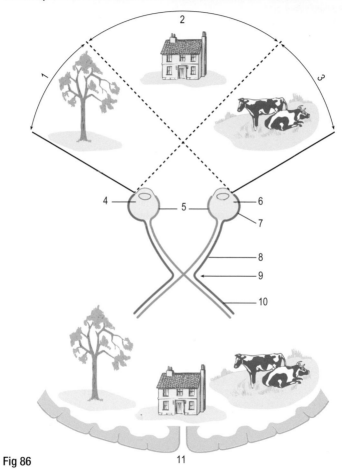

Fig 86

1. Left eye only
2. Both eyes
3. Right eye only
4. Left eye
5. Nasal retina
6. Right eye
7. Temporal retina
8. Optic nerve
9. Optic chiasma
10. Optic tract
11. Image seen by the visual centre in the occipital lobe

Comments

Physiological: Binocular vision allows one to see in three dimensions. As both eyes look at the same object, each eye sees it better on its own side, and the images overlap in the middle. These images are fused in the brain so that only one image is seen.

Clinical: Binocular vision allows one to judge the distance, depth, height, width and length of one object with respect to another.

The extrinsic ocular muscles

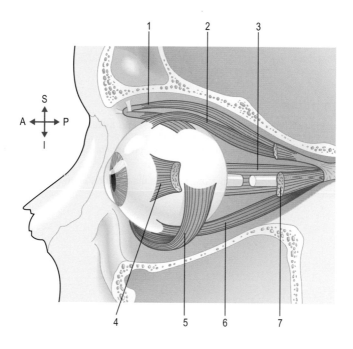

Fig 87

1. Superior oblique muscle
2. Superior rectus muscle
3. Right medial rectus muscle
4. Right lateral rectus muscle (cut)
5. Inferior oblique muscle
6. Inferior rectus muscle
7. Lateral rectus muscle (cut)

Comments

Anatomical: The extrinsic ocular muscles comprise the muscles of the eyelids and the six extraocular muscles, four rectus muscles and two oblique muscles. The medial, superior and inferior rectus muscles and the inferior oblique muscle are supplied by the 3rd cranial nerve, the superior oblique muscle by the 4th cranial nerve and the lateral rectus muscle by the 6th cranial nerve.

Physiological: The muscles mobilise and direct the eyeball as follows — the medial rectus medially, the superior rectus superiorly, the inferior rectus inferiorly and laterally, the superior oblique inferiorly and laterally and the lateral rectus laterally.

Clinical: Eye movements are under voluntary control. Accommodation for near or distance vision is involuntary. Near vision is more tiring because of the continuous use of the muscles. Paralysis of one oculomotor nerve causes diplopia (double vision).

Section of the eye and its adnexal structures

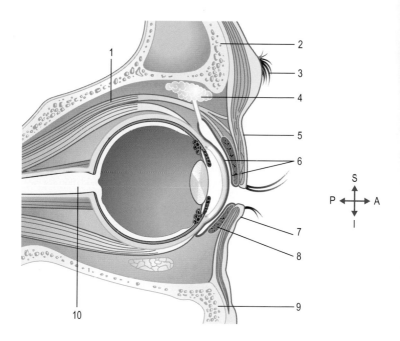

Fig 88

1. Levator palpebrae superioris muscle
2. Frontal bone
3. Eyebrow
4. Lacrimal gland
5. Upper eyelid
6. Conjunctiva
7. Lower eyelid
8. Tarsus
9. Maxillary bone
10. Optic nerve

Comments

Anatomical: The adnexal structures of the eye include the eyebrows, the eyelids, the eyelashes and the lacrimal apparatus. The eyebrows are two arched supraorbital eminences of the frontal bone covered with hairs. The eyelids are two tissue folds that cover the eye above and below and whose borders are lined by eyelashes in the form of short curved hairs. They are made up of skin, two muscles (the palpebral part of the orbicularis oculi and the levator palpebrae superioris muscle), the tarsus, which is a plate of connective tissue providing support to the other structures, and the palpebral conjunctiva. The free borders of the eyelids contain sebaceous and tarsal glands.

Physiological: These adnexal structures protect the eyes. The eyelashes protect the eyes from sweat, dust and foreign bodies. The conjunctiva protects the cornea and the anterior aspect of the eye. The tarsal glands secrete an oily fluid that coats the conjunctiva at each blink of the eye and thus prevents the tear film from evaporating. The eye is closed by contraction of the orbicularis oculi muscle. The upper eyelid is raised by contraction of the levator palpebrae superioris muscle.

Clinical: Tears and secretions regularly spread over the corneal surface, roughly every 5 seconds, as a result of blinking, which prevents it from drying. Touching the conjunctiva or the eyelashes or exposure to a bright light sets off a conjunctival reflex that closes the eye. Eye drops may be instilled into the lower conjunctival sac, which is the space lying between the lower eyelid and the eyeball.

The lacrimal apparatus

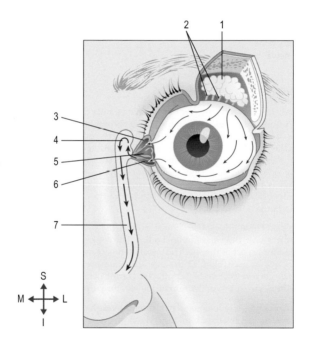

Fig 89 The *arrows* indicate the direction of flow of the tears.

1. Lacrimal gland
2. Excretory ducts of lacrimal gland
3. Upper lacrimal canaliculus
4. Lacrimal sac
5. Lacrimal caruncle
6. Lower lacrimal canaliculus
7. Nasolacrimal duct

Comments

Anatomical: In each eye, the lacrimal apparatus comprises the lacrimal gland and its excretory ducts, the two lacrimal canaliculi, the lacrimal sac and one nasolacrimal duct. The lacrimal caruncle is a reddish body separating the lacrimal canaliculi, which fuse to form the lacrimal sac.

Physiological: The lacrimal apparatus secretes and carries the tears. The exocrine lacrimal glands secrete the tears, which flow into the conjunctival sac on the eye surface and leave via the openings of the lacrimal canaliculi lining the eyelids. Tears contain water, mineral salts, antibodies and bactericidal enzymes. Tears nourish and supply the conjunctiva with oxygen, drain away waste products, prevent infections with the help of a bactericidal enzyme and keep the conjunctiva moist.

Clinical: The secretion and drainage of tears occur simultaneously. A foreign body, an irritant in the eye or emotional upset increases the secretion of tears and causes dilation of the conjunctival vessels. A dry eye syndrome due to the reduced secretion of tears can cause corneal lesions or keratitis.

The sense of smell

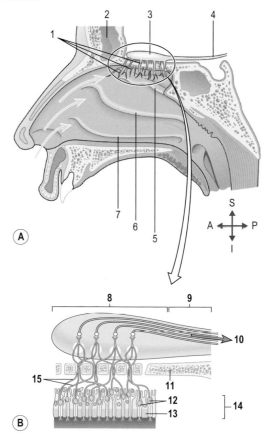

Fig 90 (A) Olfactory structures. **(B)** Magnified section of the olfactory apparatus in the nose and on the inferior surface of the brain.

1. Nerve endings and olfactory nerves
2. Frontal sinus
3. Olfactory bulb
4. Olfactory tract
5. Superior nasal concha
6. Middle nasal concha
7. Inferior nasal concha
8. Olfactory bulb
9. Olfactory tract
10. Towards the olfactory area of the temporal lobe of the brain
11. Ethmoid bone
12. Olfactory cells
13. Sustentacular cells
14. Embedded in the epithelium of the roof of the nasal cavity
15. Olfactory nerves

Comments

Anatomical: Specialised olfactory nerve endings are located in the mucosa of the roof of the nasal cavity, above the superior nasal concha.

Physiological: The sense of smell depends on the specialised olfactory nerve endings. The olfactory nerves cross the cribriform plate of the ethmoid bone, make synapses in the olfactory bulb, form the olfactory tract and enter the olfactory area in the temporal lobe of the cerebrum, which is responsible for translating the neural signals into the perception of smell.

Clinical: As a result of the process of adaptation, continuous exposure to a smell reduces perception of it. Anosmia (the loss of the sense of smell) can be caused by an inflammatory process in the nasal mucosa that prevents the odours from reaching the olfactory epithelium. Sniffing concentrates the odoriferous molecules in the nose and increases perception of them by stimulating more olfactory receptors. Smell can have an impact on taste, appetite or even the storage of olfactory memories.

The structure of the taste buds

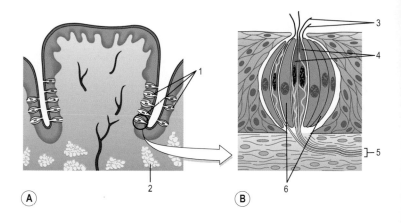

Fig 91 (A) Section of a papilla. **(B)** Magnified section of a taste bud.

1. Taste buds
2. Deep lingual glands
3. Microvilli of taste buds
4. Taste sensitive cells
5. Nerve fibres
6. Sustentacular cells

Comments

Anatomical: The taste buds are chemosensory corpuscles of the glossopharyngeal, facial and vagus nerves that are located in the epithelium of the dorsal lingual mucosa. These nerves gather to form a plexus.

Physiological: Chemical substances dissolved in saliva enter the pores of these chemosensory corpuscles, which release nerve impulses that synapse in the olfactory bulb and are then transmitted to the thalamus and the olfactory area of the parietal lobe. Smell plays a protective role against the ingestion of spoilt food.

Clinical: There are four types of taste sensation—sweet, sour, bitter and salty. The sense of taste is disrupted by a dry mouth. Taste is linked to smell, which stimulates salivation and gastric secretion.

Endocrine system

The locations of the endocrine glands

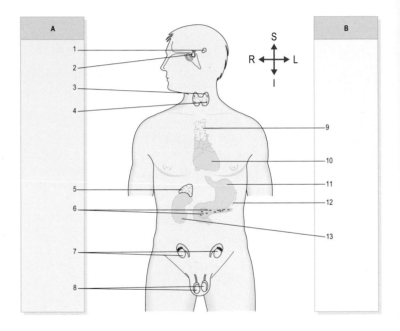

Fig 92 (A) The main endocrine glands. **(B)** Tissues and glands with secondary endocrine functions.

1. Pineal gland
2. Pituitary gland or hypophysis
3. Thyroid gland
4. Parathyroid glands (lying behind the thyroid)
5. Suprarenal gland
6. Pancreatic islets of Langerhans
7. Ovaries (in women)
8. Testes (in men)
9. Thymus
10. Heart
11. Stomach
12. Adipose tissue
13. Kidneys

Comments

Anatomical: The endocrine system is made up of numerous endocrine glands scattered throughout the body and includes the pineal gland, the pituitary gland or hypophysis, the parathyroid glands, the suprarenal glands, the pancreatic islets of Langerhans, the ovaries in women and the testes in men. These glands are physically separate—some are interrelated by the hormones that they secrete (e.g., the pituitary gland, the thyroid gland).

Physiological: The endocrine glands secrete their hormones directly into the blood. They are carried by the vascular system and, at a distance, act on specific cells to produce specific effects. A hormone can act on many cell types and can produce different effects. It is released in response to a specific stimulus that will be counteracted by a negative feedback mechanism. The stimulus for release can be its blood level or can be stimulation by another hormone secreted—for example, by the hypothalamus, which controls the pituitary gland and therefore exerts indirect effects on other glands. On reaching the target cell, the hormone binds to a specific receptor and then sets off a series of chemical or metabolic reactions within the cell. A positive feedback mechanism keeps increasing the release of the hormones until the stimulus has been blocked.

Clinical: Polyuria, polydipsia, overeating, weight loss, recurrent infections and visual disturbances are the signs and symptoms of diabetes. Facial and truncal obesity, muscle wasting, skin changes (skin striae, hirsutism, defective healing), arterial hypertension, fractures and pain are those of Cushing's syndrome.

Median section showing the location of the pituitary gland and associated structures

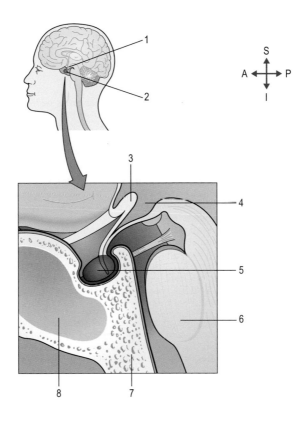

S
A ←→ P
I

1
2
3
4
5
6
7
8

Fig 93

1. Hypothalamus
2. Pituitary gland
3. Optic chiasma
4. Hypothalamus
5. Pituitary gland in the pituitary fossa
6. Pons
7. Sphenoid bone
8. Sphenoidal sinus

Comments

Anatomical: The pituitary gland lies in the sella turcica, which is a fossa in the sphenoid bone that lies below the optic chiasma. It consists of the anterior lobe (the adenohypophysis), which is an excrescence of the glandular epithelium of the pharynx, and of the posterior lobe, which is an extension of the cerebral tissue.

Physiological: The pituitary and the hypothalamus control the activity of most of the endocrine glands. The adenohypophysis secretes growth hormone and prolactin, as well as the trophic hormones that act on the other target endocrine glands, such as the thyroid (thyroid-stimulating hormone), the gonads and the suprarenal glands (adrenocorticotropic hormone [ACTH]).

Clinical: The secretion of growth hormone or somatostatin increases during adolescence and during sleep and also in response to hypoglycaemia, physical activity and anxiety. Its secretion is suppressed by hyperglycaemia or the release of gastrointestinal hormones. Hypersecretion of growth hormone occurs in acromegaly.

Pituitary gland (1): its lobes and their relations to the hypothalamus

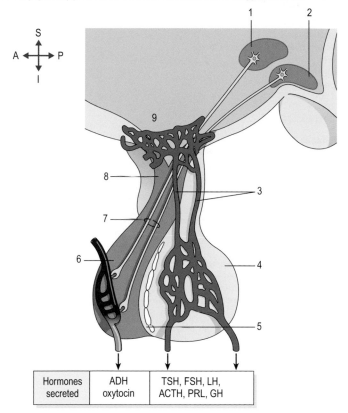

Hormones secreted	ADH oxytocin	TSH, FSH, LH, ACTH, PRL, GH

Fig 94 *ACTH,* Adrenocorticotropic hormone; *ADH,* antidiuretic hormone; *FSH,* follicle-stimulating hormone; *GH,* growth hormone; *LH,* luteinizing hormone; *PRL,* prolactin; *TSH,* thyroid-stimulating hormone.

1. Paraventricular nucleus
2. Supraoptic nucleus
3. Hypothalamohypophyseal portal system
4. Anterior lobe
5. Intermediate lobe
6. Posterior lobe
7. The hypothalamohypophyseal tract
8. Pituitary stalk
9. Third ventricle

Comments

Anatomical: The hypothalamus and the pituitary gland are linked by the pituitary stalk. There is also a portal venous system that links them and allows the transport of releasing and inhibitory hormones from the hypothalamus to the pituitary. The blood supply to the pituitary consists of a branch of the internal carotid artery and a portal venous system.

Physiological: The pituitary and the hypothalamus control the activity of most of the endocrine glands. The anterior lobe (adenohypophysis) secretes stimulating hormones that act on other target endocrine organs, such as the thyroid, the gonads and the suprarenals. Growth hormone stimulates growth by increasing cell division in bones and muscles and also stimulates protein synthesis while promoting lipid catabolism and raising the blood sugar level. Prolactin, secreted during pregnancy, promotes lactation. Thyroid-stimulating hormone stimulates the thyroid gland to secrete triiodothyronine (T_3) and thyroxine (T_4). ACTH increases the concentration of cholesterol in the suprarenal gland and the secretion of cortisol and of androgenic steroids. The gonadotrophins are FSHs (follicle-stimulating hormones), which stimulate the ovarian follicles to grow, and LHs (luteinising hormones), which luteinise the follicles. Hormonal secretion is controlled by positive or negative feedback.

Clinical: Low blood pressure, weakness, dizzy spells, pallor, depigmentation, hair loss, skin atrophy, amenorrhoea in women and impotence in men are signs and symptoms of pituitary failure. The fact that ACTH blood levels reach a maximum at 8 a.m. has an impact on the circadian rhythm throughout one's life, affecting the sleep cycle, working hours and changes in time zones. At puberty, the gonadotrophins cause maturation of the male and female sex organs.

Pituitary gland (2): synthesis and storage of the antidiuretic hormone and oxytocin

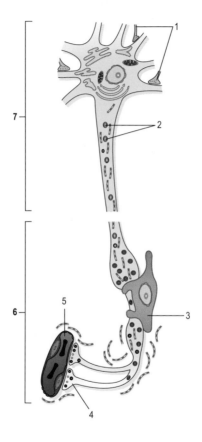

Fig 95

1. Presynaptic neurones
2. Vesicles containing the hypothalamic hormones, antidiuretic hormone and oxytocin
3. Pituicyte
4. Axon terminal
5. Capillaries in the posterior lobe
6. Posterior lobe (neurohypophysis)
7. Hypothalamus

Comments

Anatomical: The posterior lobe (the neurohypophysis) is made up of pituicytes, which are neuroglial cells that have a supporting role. The neurohypophyseal hormones are synthesised by the neurones in the hypothalamus, transported by their axons and stored in the granules in the axon terminals.

Physiological: A low blood level of one circulating hormone in the hypothalamus promotes specific secretion of the appropriate hypothalamic-releasing hormone, which is then carried down along the hypothalamohypophyseal portal system to stimulate the secretion of the appropriate hormone by the adenohypophysis. This is the mechanism of negative feedback. The neurohypophysis secretes oxytocin and antidiuretic hormone (ADH). Oxytocin and ADH are released from the axon terminals and act on nonendocrine targets. Oxytocin stimulates the smooth muscle of the uterus, as well as muscle cells in the breasts during lactation. ADH increases the water permeability of the cells of the distal convoluted tubules, the collecting ducts and the reabsorption of water.

Clinical: In cases of dehydration, the secretion of ADH is increased. A high blood level of ADH can explain the presence of reduced urine production. When very large amounts of liquid are ingested, ADH secretion is decreased.

Location of the thyroid gland and adjacent structures

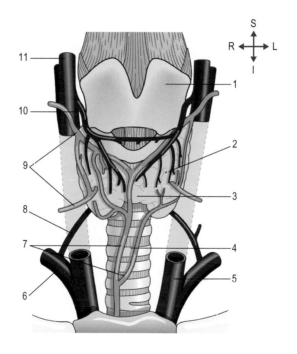

Fig 96

1. Thyroid cartilage
2. Left lobe of thyroid gland
3. Isthmus of thyroid gland
4. Trachea
5. Left common carotid artery (cut)
6. Right subclavian artery
7. Inferior thyroid veins
8. Right inferior thyroid artery
9. Veins draining into the right jugular vein
10. Right superior thyroid artery
11. Right external carotid artery

Comments

Anatomical: The thyroid gland is located in the neck, anterior to the larynx and trachea at the level of the cervical vertebrae. It has the shape of a butterfly, with two lobes linked by an isthmus. It receives a rich blood supply from the superior and inferior thyroid arteries. The thyroid veins drain into the internal jugular veins. The recurrent laryngeal nerves run close to its two lobes. The thyroid is made up of roughly spherical follicles.

Physiological: The thyroid gland secretes T_3 in larger amounts than T_4. The action of these hormones is to speed up the metabolism of muscle tissue (resulting in faster conduction in muscles, especially the myocardium); of nervous tissue (resulting in speeding up conduction and in reducing the time needed for reflex activity); and of the alimentary tract (resulting in faster transit). T_3 and T_4 also enhance the metabolism of carbohydrates, lipids, proteins and water. The parafollicular cells in the thyroid produce the hormone calcitonin.

Clinical: Tachycardia, raised body temperature, heat intolerance, excessive sweating, increased appetite, thirst, weight loss, diarrhoea and fatigability are the signs and symptoms of hyperthyroidism. An opposite set of signs and symptoms, such as cold sensitivity, weight gain and a reduced metabolic rate, suggest hypothyroidism. The onset of a goitre, associated with a variable degree of enlargement and pain and with increased prominence of the gland, is a typical feature of thyroid disease.

Location of the parathyroid glands and adjacent structures, posterior view

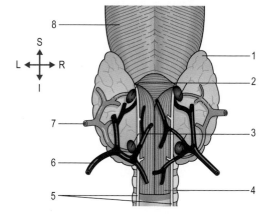

Fig 97

1. Right lobe of the thyroid
2. The two superior parathyroid glands
3. The two inferior parathyroid glands
4. Oesophagus
5. Right and left recurrent laryngeal nerves
6. Left inferior thyroid artery
7. Left middle thyroid vein
8. Pharynx

Comments

Anatomical: The parathyroid glands are small in size and are four in number, with two of them lying buried in each lobe of the thyroid gland.

Physiological: They secrete parathormone, which controls blood calcium levels; it is secreted in cases of hypocalcaemia. It increases the amount of calcium absorbed by the small intestine and reabsorbed by the renal tubules. It can also release calcium via the bone-resorbing activity of the osteoclasts. Parathormone and calcitonin also influence the activity of muscles and nerves and blood coagulation.

Clinical: Muscle cramps, potentially progressing to tetany, neuromuscular irritability and convulsions, are the signs and symptoms of hypoparathyroidism. Cardiac arrhythmia, intestinal problems (e.g., epigastric pain, nausea, vomiting, constipation), mental changes (e.g., asthenia), muscular disorders (e.g., muscle weakness, feeling of pins and needles), psychiatric disturbances, bone pain worsened by application of local pressure and repeated spontaneous fractures are the signs and symptoms of hyperparathyroidism.

Respiratory system

The structures associated with the respiratory system

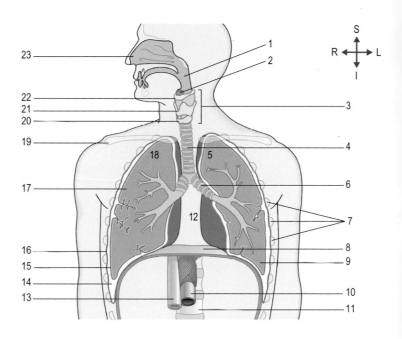

Fig 98

1. Pharynx
2. Epiglottis
3. Larynx
4. Trachea
5. Apex
6. Left main bronchus
7. Ribs
8. Diaphragm
9. Base of left lung
10. Aorta
11. Vertebral column
12. Cardiac cavity

13. Inferior vena cava
14. Pleural cavity
15. Visceral pleura
16. Parietal pleura
17. Right lung
18. Apex
19. Right clavicle
20. Cricoid cartilage
21. Thyroid cartilage
22. Hyoid bone
23. Nose

Comments

Anatomical: The organs of the respiratory system include the nose, the pharynx, the larynx, the trachea, the bronchi, the bronchioles, the two lungs and their pleural coverings, the intercostal muscles and the diaphragm.

Physiological: The chemical activity of the cells of the body needs energy and oxygen (O_2) and releases carbon dioxide (CO_2). The respiratory system consists of the structures that ensure the supply of atmospheric O_2 and the excretion of CO_2.

Clinical: The colour of the skin and of the nails provides information about the respiratory system. The skin and the nails are normally pink. Cyanosis can occur in cases of respiratory failure or airway obstruction, for example.

The constituent structures of the nasal septum

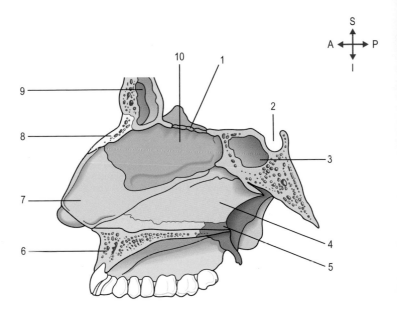

Fig 99

1. Cribriform plate of the ethmoid bone
2. Pituitary fossa
3. Sphenoidal sinus
4. Vomer
5. Palatine bone
6. Maxilla
7. Septal cartilage
8. Nasal bone
9. Frontal sinus
10. Perpendicular plate of ethmoid bone

Comments

Anatomical: The nasal septum consists, posteriorly, of the perpendicular plate of the ethmoid bone and of the vomer, anteriorly, of the septal cartilage, superiorly, of the cribriform plate of the ethmoid bone and of the sphenoid, frontal and nasal bones and inferiorly, of the maxillary and palatine bones.

Physiological: The septum separates the two nasal cavities.

Clinical: A nosebleed (epistaxis) is due to the expulsion of blood from the nasal fossae via the choanae (posterior nasal apertures). The common cold or coryza is due to a highly contagious rhinovirus and is associated with a runny nose (rhinorrhoea), sneezing, pharyngitis and a low-grade fever.

The lateral wall of the right nasal cavity

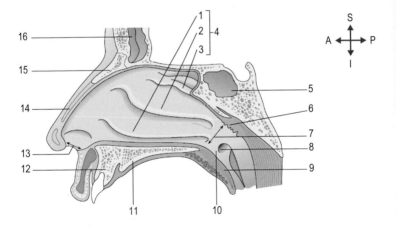

Fig 100

210

1. Inferior nasal concha
2. Middle nasal concha
3. Superior nasal concha
4. Ethmoid bone
5. Sphenoidal sinus
6. Pharyngeal tonsil
7. Posterior nasal apertures (choanae)
8. Opening of auditory (eustachian) tube
9. Soft palate
10. Nasopharynx
11. Hard palate
12. Maxilla
13. Anterior nasal apertures
14. Septal cartilage
15. Nasal bone
16. Frontal sinus

Comments

Anatomical: The nasal cavity is divided into two cavities by the septum, which acts as a partition wall and consists of the septal cartilage and the frontal and nasal bones anteriorly, of the ethmoid and sphenoid bones superiorly and of the maxillary bone and the hard palate inferiorly. It communicates with the paranasal sinuses, which are air-containing cavities inside the facial and cranial bones. The nasal cavity has hairy anterior apertures and posterior apertures connecting it with the pharynx. It is lined by a highly vascular epithelium that joins the nasal epithelium at the level of the nasopharynx.

Physiological: The nasal cavity is an airway designed to warm up, humidify, filter and clean up the inspired air and to serve as the olfactory organ. The cells of the ciliated epithelium or mucosa lining the cavity and the three conchae of the ethmoid bone, which increase the exposed surface, secrete mucus, and help warm up, humidify and filter the inspired air. The paranasal sinuses (maxillary, frontal and ethmoidal) act as resonators during speech. Smell is detected by specialised receptors, which are located in the cribriform plate of the ethmoid and in the superior nasal conchae, and which send neural signals via the olfactory nerves to the brain for decoding.

Clinical: Viral infections of the nose and of the pharynx can spread to the sinuses and be complicated by secondary bacterial infections. An acute sinusitis can recur and become chronic.

View of the passage of air from the nose to the larynx

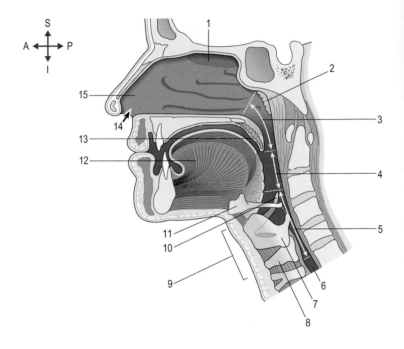

Fig 101

1. Olfactory epithelium
2. Pharyngeal tonsil
3. Nasopharynx
4. Oropharynx
5. Laryngopharynx
6. Oesophagus
7. Thyroid cartilage
8. Cricoid cartilage
9. Larynx
10. Epiglottis
11. Hyoid bone
12. Tongue
13. Soft palate and uvula
14. Air
15. Nasal cavity

Comments

Anatomical: The pharynx lies between the choanae and the larynx and is made up of three parts — the nasopharynx, the oropharynx and the laryngopharynx. The nasopharynx, posterior to the nose, contains the openings of the eustachian tubes from the middle ear and the tonsils. The oropharynx contains the palatine tonsils.

Physiological: The pharynx, which allows the passage of air and food, plays a role in both the respiratory and the alimentary systems. On its way through the nose and the mouth, the air is warmed up and humidified. During swallowing, the mucosa protects the underlying tissue from damage caused by the passage of food along the mouth and the pharynx. The lymphoid tissue in the submucosa and the tonsils protects against infection by producing antibodies. The oropharynx is important in swallowing by preventing the reflux of food into the nasal cavity. The pharyngeal muscles keep the oropharynx open to facilitate breathing and closed during swallowing. The pharynx and the paranasal sinuses act as resonators during speech.

Clinical: Every person has a characteristic voice. Snoring and sleep disorders can be caused by a loss of muscular tone, which allows the muscles and the mucosal surfaces of the throat to vibrate. Swallowing the wrong way is due to failure of closure of the larynx during swallowing.

Larynx (1), posterior view

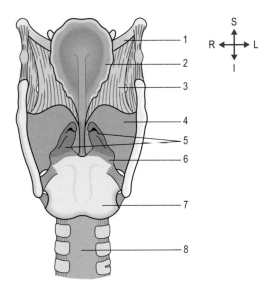

Fig 102

1. Hyoid bone
2. Epiglottis
3. Thyrohyoid membrane
4. Thyroid cartilage
5. Arytenoid cartilages
6. Cricoarytenoid ligament
7. Cricoid cartilage (its large posterior part)
8. Trachea

Comments

Anatomical: The larynx consists of the thyroid, cricoid and arytenoid cartilages and the epiglottis, all linked together by ligaments and membranes. The anterior projection of the thyroid cartilage in the throat corresponds to the laryngeal protuberance (Adam's apple). The cricoid cartilage is the posterior boundary of the upper airways. The vocal cords are attached to the arytenoid cartilages, which are hyaline cartilages, in contrast to that of the epiglottis, which is made up of fibroelastic cartilage. The laryngeal arteries and veins provide the blood supply to the larynx. It is supplied by parasympathetic fibres from the vagus nerve and by sympathetic nerves from the superior cervical ganglion.

Physiological: The larynx has a role in conveying, warming up, humidifying and filtering air and in producing sounds and protecting the airways. The epiglottis closes the larynx during swallowing.

Clinical: The larynx enlarges in men after puberty, leading to prominence of the Adam's apple and a deeper voice. The signs and symptoms of laryngopharyngeal disease include dysphagia, dysphonia, pharyngeal obstruction or pain, pain on swallowing, a feeling of the presence of a foreign body and earache.

Larynx (2), anterior view

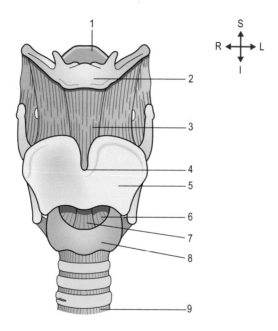

S
R ←——→ L
I

Fig 103

1. Epiglottis
2. Hyoid bone
3. Thyrohyoid membrane
4. Superior thyroid notch
5. Thyroid cartilage
6. Cricovocal membrane (conus elasticus)
7. Cricothyroid ligament
8. Cricoid cartilage (narrow anterior part)
9. Trachea

Comments

Anatomical: The larynx links the laryngopharynx to the trachea. The cricoid cartilage lies below the thyroid cartilage, which it is linked to by the cricothyroid ligament; it also overlies the larynx and articulates with the arytenoid cartilage. The epiglottis, made up of fibroelastic cartilage, is attached to the anterior wall of the thyroid cartilage.

Physiological: The epiglottis closes the larynx during swallowing, preventing any risk of inhaling food into the lungs.

Clinical: The Adam's apple, lying in front of the throat, is palpable and is much larger in postpubertal males. Coughing during eating should be a warning of the risk of food inhalation—that is, food going down the wrong way.

The cricoid cartilage, lateral view

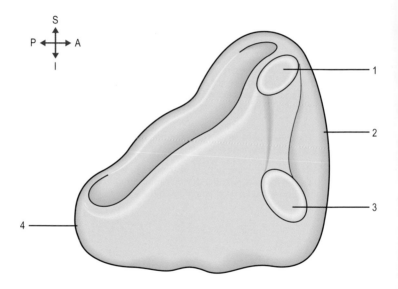

Fig 104

1. Articular facet for arytenoid cartilage
2. Large posterior aspect
3. Articular facet for thyroid artery
4. Narrow anterior aspect

Comments

Anatomical: The cricoid cartilage, consisting of hyaline cartilage, is shaped like a signet ring. It is a complete ring that hugs the larynx tightly; it is not distensible or compressible. It articulates with the thyroid and arytenoid cartilages. Its lower border is the boundary of the upper airways.

Physiological: It has a role in breathing and swallowing and allows the respiratory tract to stay open by preventing collapse of its walls.

Clinical: Asphyxia due to inhalation of food or of a foreign object is a medical emergency requiring removal of the obstruction because the walls of the respiratory tract cannot dilate to allow the passage of air.

The vocal cords

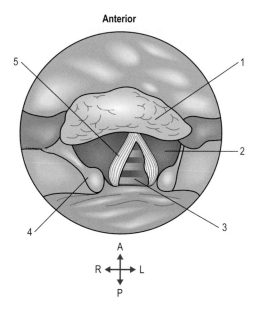

Anterior

Fig 105

220

1. Epiglottis
2. Vestibular fold
3. Trachea (with its cartilaginous rings visible)
4. Arytenoid cartilage
5. Vocal cord

Comments

Anatomical: The vocal cords are two mucosal folds with free borders, arranged in the shape of a cone and attached to the arytenoid cartilages. The glottis (rima glottidis) is the space between the vocal cords.

Physiological: The movements of the muscles controlling the vocal chords include abduction and adduction. Relaxation of the muscles allows air to enter the larynx and the vibrations of the vocal cords to produce a low note. On the other hand, when the vocal chords are tensed, the passage of air produces a high note. The volume of the voice depends on the tension of the muscles as they alter the length and degree of separation of the vocal cords and on the expiratory force. High notes are related to shorter vocal cords. Phonation depends on the actions of the lips, the tongue and the cheeks.

Clinical: A weakened voice, dysphonia (difficulty in speaking and making sounds), hoarseness, repeated throat clearing, cough and noisy breathing are possible signs and symptoms of disease of the vocal chords.

Extreme positions of the vocal cords in abduction (open)

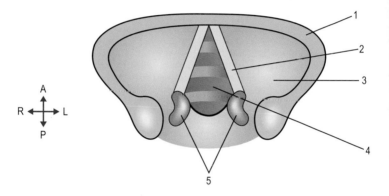

A
R ←→ L
P

Fig 106

222

1. Thyroid cartilage
2. Vocal chords
3. Vestibular fold
4. Trachea with its visible cartilaginous rings
5. Arytenoid cartilages

Comments

Anatomical: The vocal cords are two mucosal folds with free borders, arranged in the shape of a cone and attached to the arytenoid cartilages. The glottis (rima glottidis) is the space between the vocal cords.

Physiological: Abduction is a movement of the muscles that control the vocal cords. In abduction, the muscles of the vocal cords are relaxed, and the space between the cords is open, allowing the passage of air into the larynx. The vibrations of the cords produce a low-pitched sound.

Clinical: On clinical examination, the physician must observe the mobility, colour and length of the vocal cords, as well as their vibrations when vowels are pronounced.

Extreme positions of the vocal cords in adduction (closed)

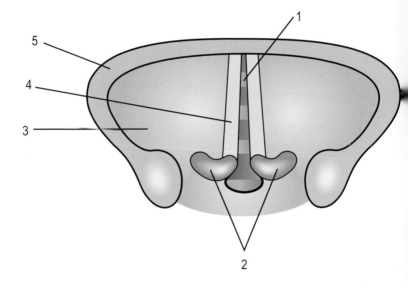

Fig 107

1. Rima glottidis
2. Arytenoid cartilages
3. Vestibular fold
4. Vocal chords
5. Thyroid cartilage

Comments

Anatomical: The vocal cords are mucosal folds, with free borders arranged in the shape of a cone, attached to the arytenoid cartilages. The glottis (rima glottidis) is the space between the vocal cords.

Physiological: Adduction is a movement of the muscles that control the vocal cords. In adduction, the muscles of the vocal cords are contracted, and the cords are tensed. The passage of air coming from the lungs produces vibrations that result in a high-pitched sound. The high pitch of the voice depends on the tension in the vocal cord muscles.

The trachea and some adjacent structures

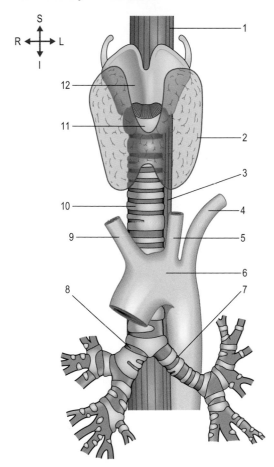

Fig 108

1. Laryngopharynx
2. Thyroid gland
3. Oesophagus
4. Left common carotid artery
5. Left subclavian artery
6. Aorta
7. Left main bronchus
8. Right main bronchus
9. Brachiocephalic trunk
10. Trachea
11. Cricoid cartilage
12. Thyroid cartilage

Comments

Anatomical: The trachea, about 10 cm long, lies anterior to the oesophagus from the level of the larynx down to the sixth thoracic vertebra. Anteriorly, its relations include the isthmus of the thyroid gland, the aortic arch and the sternum; laterally, they include the lungs and the thyroid gland. The trachea divides into two bronchi at the level of the sixth vertebra. Its blood supply depends on the inferior thyroid arteries and veins and the bronchial arteries. Its lymphatic drainage is via the paratracheal lymph nodes.

Physiological: The trachea warms, humidifies and filters the inhaled air, secretes mucus and participates in the cough reflex.

Clinical: Coughing is the reflex expulsion of inhaled particles, with or without the help of bronchial secretions. Typically, it can be acute (short-lasting) or chronic (lasting for over 1 month); it can be productive, with expectoration, or nonproductive, associated with a dry cough. It can occur at rest or with exercise, at night or during the day, and with or without exposure to environmental allergens.

The relations between the trachea and the oesophagus

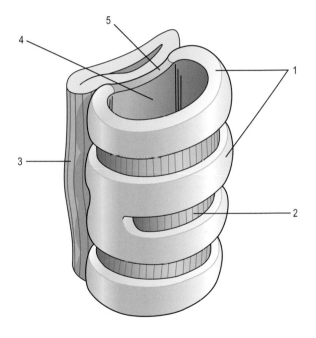

Fig 109

1. C-shaped cartilaginous rings
2. Trachea
3. Oesophagus
4. Tracheal lumen
5. Tracheal muscle

Comments

Anatomical: The trachea lies anterior to the oesophagus in the superior mediastinum. Its wall consists of three tissue layers, and it is kept open by its 20 incomplete, C-shaped, cartilaginous rings arranged in tiers.

Physiological: The cartilages maintain the patency of the trachea and its muscles control its diameter. Its parasympathetic supply comes from the recurrent nerves and the vagus nerves; when stimulated, they cause it to contract, whereas the sympathetic nerves coming from the sympathetic ganglia cause it to dilate.

Clinical: Haemoptysis is the spitting of blood that comes from the subglottic airways. It can be described in terms of its appearance, depending on the colour of the blood, and its volume can be described as light (blood-tinged sputum) or abundant. The latter case is a medical emergency because of the significant risk of bronchial obstruction and asphyxia. Haemoptysis can be associated with coughing and a metallic taste in the mouth. It can be a diagnostic sign of a bronchial cancer.

The cells lining the trachea: the ciliated mucosa

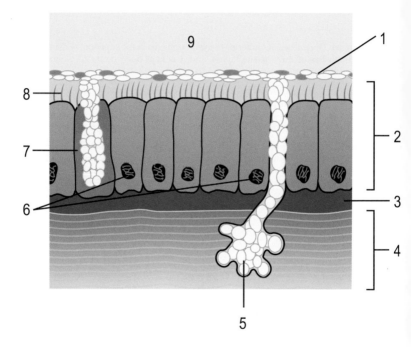

Fig 110

1. Mucus layer with entrapped particles
2. Cylindrical ciliated epithelium
3. Basement membrane
4. Submucosa
5. Mucous gland in the submucosa
6. Mucus
7. Goblet cells
8. Cilia
9. Lumen of the airway

Comments

Anatomical; Three tissue layers coat the tracheal cartilages—an internal epithelial layer, a basement membrane and a submucosal layer. The cylindrical ciliated epithelium also contains goblet cells.

Physiological: The goblet cells secrete mucus.

Clinical: Smoking causes a progressive loss of the ciliated cells.

Organs related to the lungs

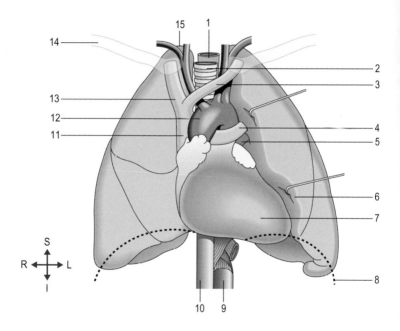

Fig 111

1. Oesophagus
2. Trachea
3. Left brachiocephalic vein
4. Pulmonary artery
5. One left pulmonary vein
6. Left lung (retracted)
7. Heart
8. Diaphragm

9. Aorta
10. Inferior vena cava
11. Superior vena cava
12. Aorta
13. Right brachiocephalic vein
14. Clavicle
15. Pulmonary apex

Comments

Anatomical: There are two lungs, with each lung having a costal surface and a medial surface, an apex and a base. The lateral surfaces of the lungs are in contact with the ribs, the costal cartilages and the intercostal muscles. Their medial surfaces enclose the space between the lungs—the mediastinum, which contains the large vessels, lymphatics, nerves, the trachea and the two main bronchi, right and left. The base of the lung lies in the thoracic cavity close to the diaphragm; the apex lies at the root of the neck close to the clavicle, the ribs, some blood vessels and some nerves.

Physiological: The diaphragm is a respiratory muscle, along with the 11 pairs of intercostal muscles. Inspiratory expansion of the thorax is under voluntary and involuntary control.

Clinical: The respiratory rate is the number of inspiratory and expiratory cycles per minute. It is measured by watching the movements of the diaphragm. The normal rate varies with age and decreases as one ages. It is about 40 to 60 cycles per minute in neonates and 14 to 16 in adults. A lower rate and a higher rate correspond to bradypnoea and tachypnoea, respectively. The expiratory phase is about 1.5 times longer than the inspiratory phase. The respiratory rate increases adaptively with stress or physical activity, and it decreases during sleep. An abnormality in this rate indicates some form of respiratory distress.

The pulmonary lobes and the blood vessels and airways of each lobe, medial views

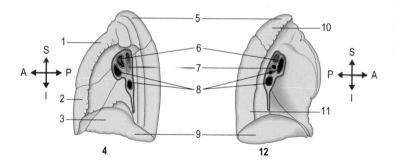

Fig 112

1. Upper lobe
2. Middle lobe
3. Lower lobe
4. Right lung
5. Apices (right and left)
6. Pulmonary arteries (right and left)
7. Main bronchi (right and left)
8. Pulmonary veins (right and left)
9. Bases (right and left)
10. Upper lobe
11. Lower lobe
12. Left lung

Comments

Anatomical: The right lung has three lobes — upper, middle and lower — whereas the left lung has only two lobes, upper and middle. Each lobe has many lobules. At the level of the fifth thoracic vertebra, the trachea branches into the main right and left bronchi.

Physiological: The bronchi are conducting structures that carry air into the lungs, where gas exchange occurs in the alveoli.

Clinical: By examining the appearance and colour of the skin, one can judge whether the respiratory system is in good shape. Cyanosis of the lips and nails is a sign of hypoxia. Dyspnoea, spitting of phlegm, coughing, haemoptysis, copious purulent expectoration and chest pain are signs and symptoms of respiratory disease.

The relations of the pleura and of the lungs

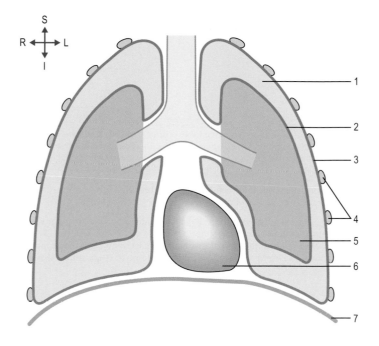

S
R ←→ L
I

1
2
3
4
5
6
7

Fig 113

1. Pleural cavity with serous fluid
2. Visceral pleura
3. Parietal pleura
4. Ribs
5. Lung
6. Heart
7. Diaphragm

Comments

Anatomical: Each lung is surrounded by its pleura, which is a serous membrane with two layers. The visceral layer is adherent to the lung; the parietal layer is adherent to the thoracic wall and the diaphragm. In the mediastinum, at the hilum of the lung, both layers become continuous. Between these two layers, there is some serous fluid secreted in small quantities by the epithelial cells of the membrane.

Physiological: The serous fluid prevents these layers from sticking to each other and allows them to slide past each other during breathing.

Clinical: Respiratory distress suggests the introduction of air or fluid into the pleural sacs. Dyspnoea, pain and coughing are signs and symptoms of pleural effusion.

The flow of blood between the heart and the lungs

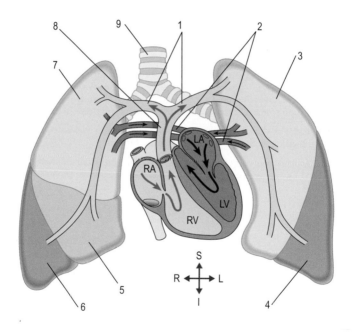

Fig 114 *LA,* Left atrium; *LV,* left ventricle; *RA,* right atrium; *RV,* right ventrivcle.

1. Right and left pulmonary arteries
2. Pulmonary veins
3. Upper lobe
4. Lower lobe
5. Middle lobe
6. Lower lobe
7. Upper lobe
8. Pulmonary trunk
9. Trachea

Comments

Anatomical: The pulmonary trunk bifurcates into the right and left pulmonary arteries, which divide further to transport deoxygenated blood through each lung, down to the capillaries in the alveolar walls. The pulmonary capillaries unite to form the pulmonary venules, which also unite to form the two pulmonary veins. The oxygenated blood is then transported to the left atrium.

Physiological: Gas exchange takes place across the walls of the capillaries and the alveoli.

Clinical: A sudden pain in the chest coupled with dyspnoea and a predisposing clinical context (e.g., prolonged confinement to bed, postpartum state, advanced progressive cancer) must raise the suspicion of a pulmonary embolus causing obstruction of a pulmonary artery or its branches. This must be followed by an examination of the lower limb looking for a veinous thrombus, which could be the source of the embolus. A massive pulmonary embolus can be fatal.

The lower airways

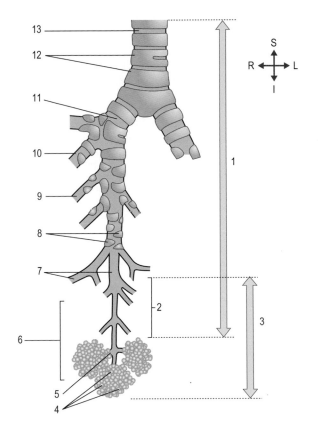

Fig 115

1. The pathway of air
2. Respiratory bronchioles
3. Site of gas exchange
4. Alveoli
5. Alveolar duct
6. Lobule
7. Bronchioles
8. Bronchial cartilage
9. Segmental bronchus
10. Lobar bronchus
11. Main bronchus
12. Cartilaginous rings
13. Trachea

Comments

Anatomical: The trachea divides into two main branches, one for the right and the other for the left lung. The right main bronchus enters the lung at the hilum. It is large, short and vertically oriented, and it subdivides into three branches, each of which goes to one of the lobes before dividing into the bronchioles, the terminal bronchioles and the alveolar ducts, which break up into the alveoli. The left bronchus behaves similarly, except that it divides into two branches, with each going to one of its two lobes.

Physiological: The airways conduct air into the lungs, but gas exchange occurs only at the alveolar level. The speed and the quantity of airflow to the lungs are controlled by the contraction or relaxation of the smooth muscles in the bronchial walls.

Clinical: The risk of inhalation is greater in the right main bronchus because of its anatomical peculiarity. As a result, pulmonary diseases following inhalation are more frequent on the right side.

The alveoli and their capillary plexuses (1): group of intact alveoli

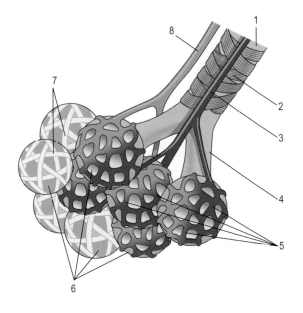

Fig 116

1. Respiratory bronchiole
2. Smooth muscle
3. Venule draining towards the pulmonary vein
4. Alveolar duct
5. Capillaries
6. Alveoli
7. Elastic fibres
8. Arteriole (coming from the pulmonary artery)

Comments

Anatomical: As they divide, the airways become progressively smaller, to the point of containing only a single epithelial layer in the alveolar ducts and the alveoli. Gas exchange occurs across the respiratory surfaces formed by the membranes of 150 million alveolar sacs clustered in close contact with the membranes of the capillaries.

Physiological: Their epithelial cells secrete a liquid surfactant that promotes expansion of the lungs at birth and, later in life, prevents desiccation and collapse of the alveolar walls during expiration.

Clinical: Pallor, fatigue and dyspnoea are potential indicators of pulmonary emphysema, which is the result of dilation of the alveoli, caused by progressive destruction of their elastic support. This is responsible for the decrease in the area available for gas exchange.

The alveoli and their capillary plexuses (2): section of an alveolus

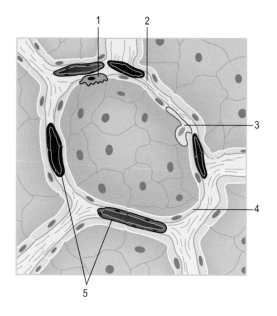

Fig 117

1. Type II pneumocyte
2. Connective tissue with elastic fibres
3. Alveolar macrophage
4. Type I pneumocyte
5. Blood capillaries

Comments

Anatomical: The alveoli are surrounded by numerous capillaries. The distal airways consist of connective tissue filled with blood and lymph capillaries, nerves, macrophages and fibroblasts. The type II pneumocytes are inserted among the type I pneumocytes and secrete surfactant.

Physiological: Surfactant secretion begins at about the 35th week of gestation and allows the lungs to expand and initiate respiration at birth.

Clinical: Premature infants are prone to respiratory failure because of a lack of surfactant, secondary to pulmonary immaturity.

The intercostal muscles and the bones of the thorax

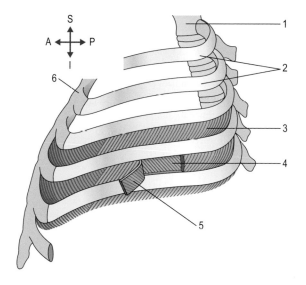

Fig 118

246

1. Vertebral column
2. Ribs
3. External intercostal muscle
4. Internal intercostal muscle
5. Internal intercostal muscle folded forward
6. Sternum

Comments

Anatomical: There are 11 pairs of muscles inserted among 12 pairs of ribs in two layers, one external and the other internal. These muscles are supplied by the intercostal nerves.

Physiological: The external intercostal muscles, directed forwards and downwards, participate in inspiration. Along with the diaphragm, they are the main inspiratory muscles. The internal intercostal muscles, directed backwards and downwards, are active during normal expiration.

Clinical: Clinically, respiration is assessed by observing or investigating its parameters at rest or during breathing. These include the respiratory rate, the degree of expansion of the thoracic cavity, any asymmetry in the elevation of the diaphragm, the type of breathing used (thoracic or abdominal), dyspnoea, abnormal in-drawing of the thoracic wall on inspiration, cyanosis and painful breathing. Cyanosis is indicated by the bluish discolouration of the integumentary system, notably the tips of the fingers and the nails. Dyspnoea is a functional indicator of the gap between respiratory needs and respiratory efficiency. Clinically, the individual is out of breath and has difficulty breathing. Dyspnoea can be graded according to the following:

a. The response to exercise—heavy exercise, walking up a slope, walking on the flat, light exercise
b. Its relationship to the respiratory cycle—during inspiration or expiration
c. The position of the patient—lying down in cases of orthopnoea and in the sitting position
d. The mode of onset—sudden or slow
e. Its periodicity and its clinical context

Dyspnoea can be caused not only by respiratory but also by cardiac or muscular problems.

The diaphragm

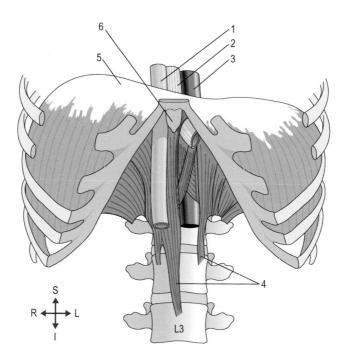

S
R ← → L
I

L3

Fig 119

1. Inferior vena cava
2. Oesophagus
3. Aorta
4. Crura of the diaphragm
5. Central tendon
6. Xiphoid process of the sternum

Comments

Anatomical: The diaphragm is a dome-shaped muscle that separates the thoracic and abdominal cavities and is supplied by the phrenic nerve. It consists of a central tendon from which muscle fibres arise on their way to their costal insertions.

Physiological: The respiratory cycle is composed of three phases — inspiration, expiration and a pause — which are repeated with the start of each new cycle. Inspiration follows contraction of the diaphragm, which reduces the intrathoracic pressure while increasing the intraabdominal pressure, and also by contraction of the external intercostal muscles. At rest, the diaphragm accounts for 75% of breathing.

Clinical: At rest, inspiration lasts for 2 to 3 seconds. The normal respiratory rate is about 15 cycles per minute. The depth of breathing is related to the excursion of the diaphragm. A diaphragmatic lesion can lead to respiratory arrest in the absence of assisted ventilation.

Changes in chest size during breathing

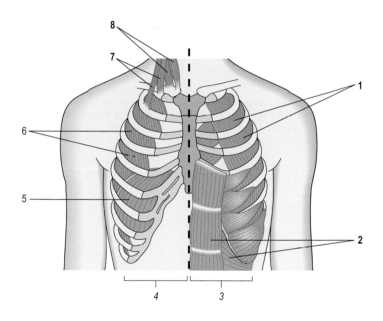

Fig 120 Muscles involved in breathing.

1. Internal intercostal muscles
2. Abdominal muscles
3. Expiration
4. Inspiration
5. Diaphragm
6. External intercostal muscles
7. Scalene muscles
8. Sternocleidomastoid muscles

Comments

Anatomical: The sternocleidomastoid and the scalene muscles extend from the vertebrae to the first ribs.

Physiological: Inspiration is an active process; expiration is a passive process. Whereas these are alternating processes, there is a continuous process of gas exchange at the alveolar level. The diffusion of O_2 and CO_2 depends on pressure differences between the atmosphere and the blood and between the blood and the tissues. The external intercostals and the diaphragm are the main muscles responsible for inspiration and expiration. During forced inspiration, the sternocleidomastoid and the scalene muscles expand the thoracic cage further as they alter the intrathoracic pressure.

Clinical: The descriptive parameters of breathing include the depth, the frequency and the rhythm of the movements involved, as well as the respiratory efforts required.

Changes in chest size during breathing, inspiratory phase

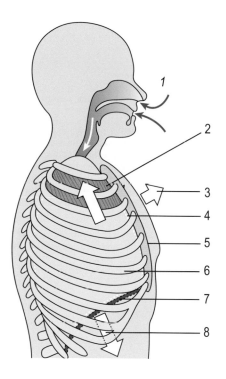

Fig 121 Changes in the thoracic volume.

1. Inspiration
2. Contraction of the external intercostal muscles
3. Distention of the thorax
4. Lung
5. Sternum
6. Rib
7. Diaphragm
8. Contraction of the diaphragm

Comments

Physiological: The volume of the thoracic cage increases with each inspiration, in accordance with the passage of air into the airways, and decreases with each expiration as the air is expelled. Inspiration is an active process during which the pulmonary tissue is stretched by the contraction of the external intercostal muscles and the diaphragm. The thoracic cage is distended, the lungs are expanded and the intraalveolar pressure drops, drawing in air to offset this drop in pressure. Meanwhile, the gas exchange occurs without interruption. This contraction of the muscles uses up energy and promotes venous return to the heart.

Clinical: The regular alternating movements of inspiration and expiration determine the respiratory rate, between 12 and 15 breaths per minute. The volume of air inspired during normal breathing, during 2 to 3 seconds, is about 500 mL. Inspiration can be forced. During forced inspiration following normal inspiration, the extra volume of air inspired is about 2.5 L. The volume of air displaced during a forced inspiration is about 5 L, equivalent to the total pulmonary capacity.

Changes in chest size during breathing, expiratory phase

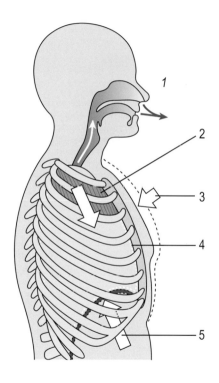

Fig 122 Changes in the thoracic volume.

1. Expiration
2. Relaxation of the external intercostal muscles
3. Collapse of the thorax
4. Lung
5. Relaxation of the diaphragm

Comments

Physiological: The volume of the thoracic cage increases with each inspiration in accordance with the passage of air into the airways and decreases with each expiration as the air is expelled. Expiration is a passive process following relaxation of the external intercostals and the diaphragm. The thorax collapses on itself as the intrapulmonary pressure rises and expels the air via the airways. Meanwhile, the gas exchange continues without interruption.

Clinical: The alternating movements of inspiration and expiration set the respiratory rate. Forced expiration can take place. The volume of air expelled during a normal expiration is about 1 L. Following quiet expiration, the volume of air contained in the trachea and bronchi, without collapse of the latter, is 150 mL. This is known as the *residual functional capacity*.

External respiration

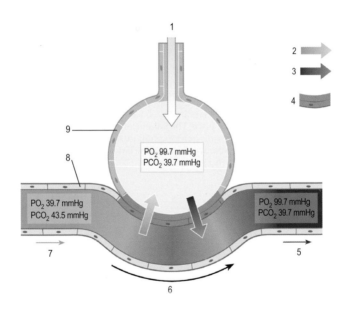

PO₂ 99.7 mmHg
PCO₂ 39.7 mmHg

PO₂ 39.7 mmHg
PCO₂ 43.5 mmHg

PO₂ 99.7 mmHg
PCO₂ 39.7 mmHg

Fig 123 *PO₂,* Partial pressure of O₂; *PCO₂,* Partial pressure of CO₂.

1. Atmospheric air
2. CO_2 movement
3. O_2 movement
4. Respiratory membrane
5. Towards the pulmonary vein
6. Direction of blood flow
7. From the pulmonary artery
8. Capillary wall
9. Alveolar wall

Comments

Physiological: This process depends on diffusional gas exchange between the alveolar sacs and the capillaries in the alveolar walls via the respiratory membranes. The deoxygenated blood entering the lungs is rich in CO_2 and poor in O_2. These two gases diffuse until their transmembrane partial pressure differences are cancelled. When the blood leaves the alveoli, the intracapillary concentration of these gases is in equilibrium with their intraalveolar concentration.

Clinical: The various forms of postinflammatory pulmonary fibrosis have multiple causes, including drugs, inhaled contaminants from mouldy hay (farmer's lung) and diffuse inflammatory diseases, such as sarcoidosis. Right from the start, these diseases alter gas exchange and diffusion by reducing the permeability and increasing the thickness of the alveolocapillary membrane.

Intratissular gas exchange

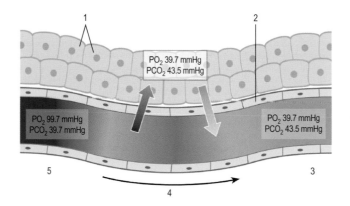

Fig 124

1. Cells in the tissues
2. Capillary wall
3. Venous end of the capillary
4. Direction of blood flow
5. Arterial end of the capillary

Comments

Physiological: This gas exchange occurs between the blood in the capillaries and the cells in the tissues. The total surface area of the intraalveolar respiratory membrane for gas exchange is almost equal to that of a tennis court. When it reaches the tissues the blood is rich in O_2 and poor in CO_2. The partial pressure of O_2 is higher in the blood than in the tissues, whereas that of CO_2 is lower. This pressure difference promotes the exchange of these gases. CO_2 diffuses out of the cell to enter the blood in the capillaries.

Clinical: Intratissular gas exchange is altered in cases of shock because of the fall in circulating blood volume, arterial blood pressure and cardiac output, resulting in the failure of hypoxic cells to satisfy their metabolic needs.

Intrapulmonary gas exchange and intratissular gas exchange

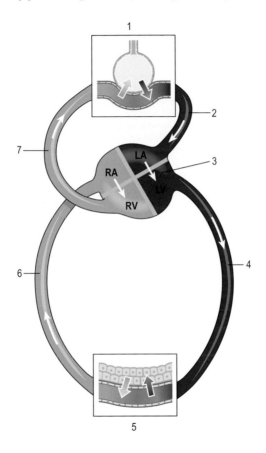

Fig 125

1. Intrapulmonary gas exchange
2. Pulmonary veins
3. Heart
4. Systemic arteries
5. Intratissular gas exchange
6. Systemic veins
7. Pulmonary arteries

LA. Left atrium
LV. Left ventricle
RV. Right ventricle
RA. Right atrium

Comments

Anatomical: The pulmonary alveolus is the anatomical unit of gas exchange. During normal breathing not all the alveoli are ventilated: those of the upper lobes are filled while the others are collapsed for the time being and their vascular perfusion is reduced.

Physiological: O_2 and CO_2 are transported in the blood. O_2 combines with haemoglobin to form oxyhaemoglobin or is dissolved in the plasma. CO_2 is diluted in the blood by the formation of bicarbonate ions or its combination to form carboxyhaemoglobin in the erythrocytes. Gas exchange depends on diffusion of the gases from a higher to a lower concentration. During intrapulmonary gas exchange, the deoxygenated blood coming to the lungs has a high partial pressure of CO_2 and a low partial pressure of O_2. These two gases diffuse according to their pressure gradients so that their concentrations in the capillaries leaving the alveoli match their intraalveolar concentrations. During intratissular gas exchange, the partial pressure of O_2 in the blood is higher than that in the tissues and vice versa for CO_2. Thus, CO_2 diffuses out of the cells to enter the blood in the capillaries, whereas O_2 diffuses into the tissues. This intratissular process supplies the cells of the body with O_2.

Clinical: The average respiratory rate is about 12 to 15 breaths per minute. The tidal volume is the volume of air inspired or expired with each normal breath and is 500 mL at rest. When there is need for more air, the tidal volume increases by recruiting more active alveoli, thus increasing intraalveolar perfusion with the blood.

Some structures involved in the control of breathing

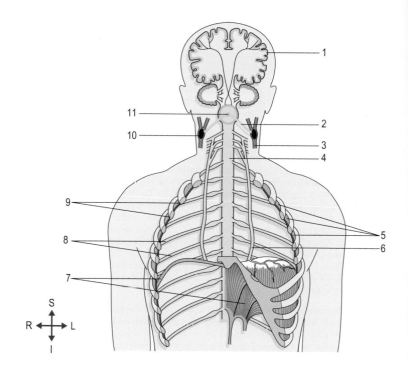

Fig 126

1. Cerebral cortex
2. Glossopharyngeal nerve
3. Carotid artery
4. Spinal cord
5. Intercostal muscles
6. Phrenic nerve for the diaphragm
7. Diaphragm
8. Intercostal nerves for the intercostal muscles
9. Cut extremities of the ribs
10. Carotid body
11. Respiratory centre in the medulla oblongata

Comments

Anatomical: The respiratory centre in the medulla oblongata consists of inspiratory neurones that actively control the frequency and depth of breathing. The nerve signals carried by the phrenic and the intercostal nerves stimulate breathing by acting on the diaphragm and the intercostal muscles.

Physiological: The control of breathing is normally involuntary but becomes voluntary during certain activities, such as singing or speaking.

Clinical: In a conscious person with hypercapnia, there is no more voluntary control of breathing; the respiratory rate is increased to augment the rate of gas exchange and reduce the partial pressure of CO_2. The normal arterial partial pressure of O_2 is between 80 and 100 mmHg, and respiratory insufficiency is diagnosed when this pressure falls below 70 mmHg. The normal arterial partial pressure of CO_2 is between 38 and 42 mmHg, and alveolar hypoventilation is diagnosed when this pressure rises above 45 mmHg.

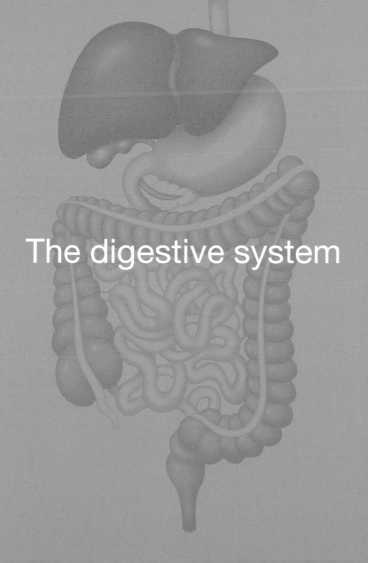

The digestive system

The digestive system

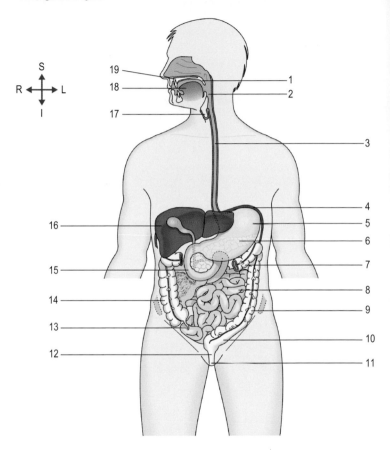

Fig 127

1. Soft palate
2. Oropharynx
3. Oesophagus
4. Diaphragm
5. Stomach
6. Pancreas (behind the stomach)
7. Transverse colon (cut)
8. Small intestine
9. Descending colon
10. Sigmoid colon
11. Anus
12. Rectum
13. Appendix
14. Ascending colon
15. Duodenum
16. Liver and gall bladder (raised)
17. Larynx
18. Tongue
19. Hard palate

Comments

Anatomical: The alimentary tract is a long tube stretching from the mouth to the anus. Food passes along this gastrointestinal tract, which is made up of organs with different functions.

Physiological: The five actions of the alimentary tract include ingestion, propulsion, digestion, absorption and excretion.

Clinical: Digestive problems suggestive of a significant lesion in an organ of the alimentary tract include bleeding, dysphagia, abdominal pain, chronic diarrhoea, bloating, constipation and complete cessation of bowel movements and the passage of flatus.

General structure of the gastrointestinal tract

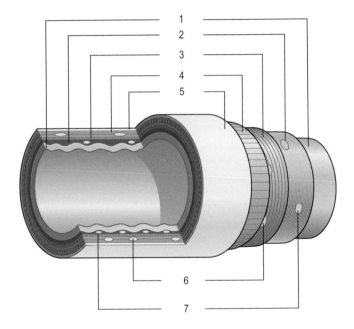

Fig 128

1. Mucosa
2. Submucosa
3. Circular muscle coat
4. Longitudinal muscle coat
5. Peritoneum
6. Myenteric plexus
7. Submucosal plexus

Comments

Anatomical: The alimentary tract from the oesophagus down exhibits a basic structural plan with a serosa or adventitia, muscularis, submucosa and mucosa, with regional modifications. In the thorax, the adventitia is made up of fibrous tissue. In the abdomen, the organs are covered by the peritoneum, which is a closed sac containing a small amount of fluid and lined by a visceral layer and a parietal layer. The muscularis consists of smooth muscle, lymphatics and blood vessels and a myenteric plexus. The submucosa is made up of connective tissue, elastic tissue, lymphoid tissue and a submucosal plexus. The two plexuses (myenteric and submucosal) are networks of sympathetic and parasympathetic nerve fibres. The mucosa consists of three layers, the mucous membrane, the lamina propria and the muscularis mucosae.

Physiological: The peritoneum protects the organs it covers from local infections and their spread. Contractions of the muscular coat, occurring in waves and controlled by the sympathetic and parasympathetic nerves, are responsible for peristaltic movements, which promote the passage of nutrients and their interactions with the digestive juices, as well as the control of the rate of digestion. The contraction of the sphincters, which are circular rings of muscle, controls the propulsion of contents and prevents reflux from occurring. The mucous membrane acts as a protective, secretory and absorptive layer.

Clinical: The peritoneum protects against the spread of infection to other organs, as in the case of appendicitis.

The peritoneal cavity, the abdominal organs of the digestive system and the pelvic organs

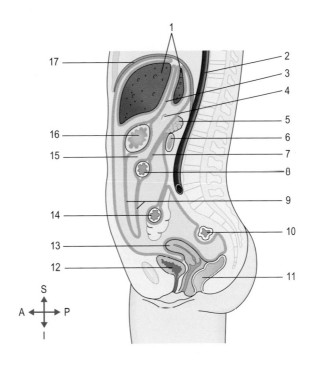

Fig 129 The peritoneal cavity is in *yellow*.

1. Liver
2. Aorta
3. Lesser omentum
4. Epiploic foramen
5. Pancreas
6. Duodenum
7. Mesentery
8. Transverse colon
9. Greater omentum
10. Sigmoid colon
11. Rectum
12. Bladder
13. Uterus
14. Small intestine
15. Lesser sac
16. Stomach
17. Diaphragm

Comments

Anatomical: The peritoneum, which is a closed sac within the abdominal cavity, has a rich vascular and lymphatic supply and contains a small amount of serous fluid between its parietal and visceral layers. The parietal layer coats the wall of the abdominal cavity and the visceral layer coats the abdominal and pelvic organs. These organs invaginate the visceral peritoneum, becoming folded on themselves and forming subperitoneal spaces.

Physiological: The peritoneum forms a protective wall against the spread of infection. The greater omentum, in the shape of an apron, is a double-layered peritoneal fold that encloses the stomach, acts as an insulator and allows the storage of fat as a source of energy.

Clinical: An abdominal pain of rapid onset, exacerbated by movement, a rise in temperature, heart rate and blood pressure, general malaise, vomiting and diarrhoea or ileus, fatigue and abdominal guarding are possible signs and symptoms of acute peritonitis. Evisceration is the extrusion of an abdominal organ via a wound or a hernia through the abdominal wall.

The greater omentum

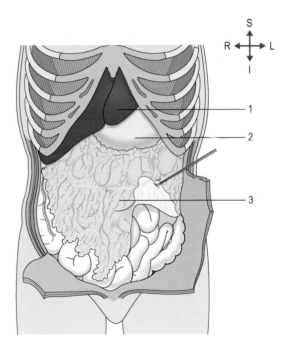

1

2

3

Fig 130

1. Liver
2. Stomach
3. Greater omentum

Comments

Anatomical: The greater omentum is an apron-like structure extending from the stomach to the colon. It is the largest peritoneal fold and is a double-layered, intraabdominal membrane. One layer covers the inner wall of the abdominal cavity, and the other covers the surface of the abdominal organs. It contains fatty tissue supplied by the gastroepiploic arteries.

Physiological: The greater omentum plays a protective role in the defence of the entire abdominopelvic cavity and has a nutritive role by storing fat for the supply of energy.

Clinical: The greater omentum is also an anatomical landmark dividing the abdominal cavity into three distinct compartments—the supramesocolic (above the transverse mesocolon), the inframesocolic (below the transverse mesocolon) and the pelvic compartments. In the inframesocolic compartment, it overlies the jejunum and the ileum. Its function is to prevent the spread of localised intraperitoneal infections or inflammatory processes, such as peritonitis.

Peristaltic movement of a bolus

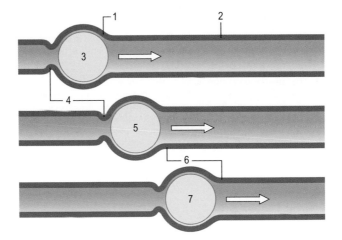

Fig 131

1. Relaxation
2. Layer of smooth muscle in the wall
3. Bolus
4. Contraction
5. Bolus
6. Relaxation
7. Bolus

Comments

Anatomical: The muscularis consists of two layers of smooth muscle traversed by blood vessels, lymphatics, and sympathetic and parasympathetic nerves.

Physiological: Contraction of the smooth muscle under the control of the sympathetic and parasympathetic nerves propels the intestinal contents forwards. Contraction of the sphincters, which are circular rings of muscle, controls the function of the alimentary tract by promoting the phases of digestion and absorption.

Clinical: A decrease or an increase in peristaltic activity is due to the stimulation of the sympathetic and parasympathetic nerves, respectively.

The cylindrical epithelium with its goblet cells

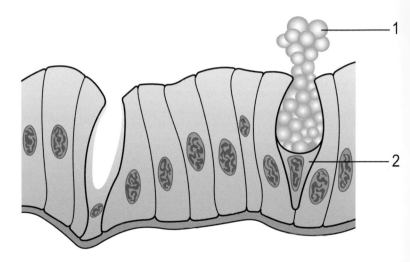

Fig 132

1. Mucus
2. Goblet cell

Comments

Anatomical: The mucosal lining of the basic wall of the alimentary tract is of two types. The first is a stratified squamous epithelium containing superficial mucous glands for the parts of the tract subjected to wear and tear; the second is a cylindrical epithelium with mucus-secreting goblet cells for the parts of the tract secreting or absorbing digestive juices and exposed to soft and moist foods.

Physiological: The mucus lubricates the walls of the tract and protects it from the damaging effects of the digestive enzymes and juices involved in the chemical breakdown of food, such as saliva, gastric juice, intestinal and pancreatic secretions and bile. It also protects against bacteria with the help of the subepithelial lymphoid tissue.

Structures visible with the mouth wide open

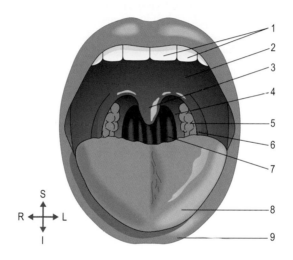

S
R ↔ L
I

1
2
3
4
5
6
7
8
9

Fig 133

1. Teeth
2. Soft palate
3. Uvula
4. Palatopharyngeal arch
5. Palatine tonsil
6. Palatoglossal arch
7. Posterior part of the pharynx
8. Tongue
9. Lower lip

Comments

Anatomical: The mouth is bordered by muscles, bones, the lips, the cheek muscles, the tongue and soft tissues of the mouth, the soft palate and the hard palate. The palate has two parts—anteriorly, a hard palate derived from the maxillary and palatine bones, and posteriorly, the soft palate, made up of a muscular component extending to the pharynx. The uvula is a membranous fold covered by a mucous membrane and giving rise to two membranous arches, the palatopharyngeal and the palatoglossal arches. The base of the tongue is tethered to the floor of the mouth, and its body tapers towards its apex. The body of the tongue is freely mobile inside the mouth.

Physiological: The buccal cavity takes part in digestion even before swallowing occurs. It receives the food, which is chewed and mixed with saliva. The taste buds embedded in the tongue allow the detection of different types of taste sensations. The tongue is involved in the tasting, chewing and swallowing of food and also in phonation. The buccal cavity plays an important role in breathing, talking, ingesting fluids, displaying facial expressions and in social interactions.

Clinical: The potential signs and symptoms of diseases of the buccal cavity include the following:

1. Bleeding and formation of white plaques (leukoplakia), red plaques (erythroplakia) and red and white plaques (erythroleukoplakia)
2. Pain, an ulcer or a chronic lesion
3. Loss of sensation or difficulty in articulating
4. Thickening of a cheek
5. Teeth or dentures that move
6. Swelling of the jaw, the salivary glands, the lymph nodes in the neck, and a tumour

Other signs include trismus (inability to open the mouth completely), pain and difficulty on swallowing or chewing.

Inferior surface of the tongue

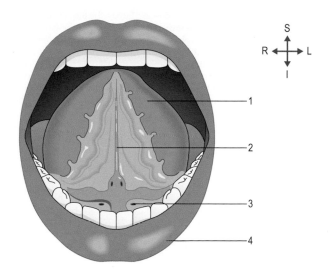

Fig 134

1. Inferior surface of the tongue
2. Frenulum of the tongue
3. Duct of salivary gland
4. Lower lip

Comments

Anatomical: The tongue is a voluntary muscle, with its surface studded with papillae that contain nerve endings of the seventh and ninth cranial nerves and function as taste receptors. It is supplied by the lingual artery and the lingual vein, which drains into the internal jugular vein. Its sensory nerve is the trigeminal (cranial nerve V), and its motor nerve is the hypoglossal nerve (cranial nerve XII). It is divided into two muscular layers, the intrinsic muscles forming the tongue itself and its extrinsic muscles. The tongue contains many parts; its base is attached to the floor of the mouth, and its body tapers towards its apex. The frenulum is a fold of its inferior mucous membrane that attaches it to the floor of the mouth. On either side of the frenulum are located the openings of the two submandibular salivary glands.

Physiological: The tongue plays a role in tasting ingested foods, phonation, chewing and swallowing. The tongue moves the unchewed food under the molars to allow it to be chewed and mixes the saliva with the food. The extrinsic muscles allow the tongue to change its position, be pulled in or stuck out and be moved from side to side. The salivary glands secrete saliva into their ducts, which drain into the mouth.

Clinical: Thrush is a fungal infection caused by *Candida albicans*, and it is associated with the formation of white plaques on the tongue and the buccal mucosa. It can strike breast-fed babies and adults suffering from a depressed immune system due to chemotherapy, as for cancer, or antibiotic therapy.

The permanent teeth and the bones of the jaw

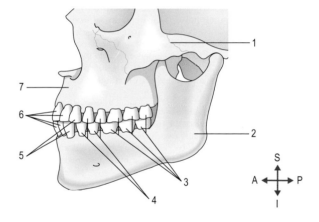

Fig 135

1. Temporomandibular joint
2. Mandible
3. Molars
4. Premolars
5. Canines
6. Incisors
7. Maxilla

Comments

Anatomical: The teeth lie in the alveolar margins of the maxilla (the upper jaw) and the mandible (the lower jaw). All the teeth have the same structure. Both the lower and the upper jaws have the same set of permanent teeth—two canines, four incisors, four premolars and six molars.

Physiological: The teeth have different shapes, depending on their functions. The incisors and the canines bite into and cut the food; the premolars and the molars crush and chew it. Their blood supply comes from the maxillary arteries and drains into the veins that join the internal jugular veins. Their nerve supply comes from the maxillary and mandibular nerves derived from the trigeminal nerve (cranial nerve V).

Clinical: Signs and symptoms of a dental abscess include pain, a localised dome-like swelling, reddening of the gum, the presence of pus released under pressure, mobility of one tooth and a swollen submandibular lymph node.

The roof of the mouth

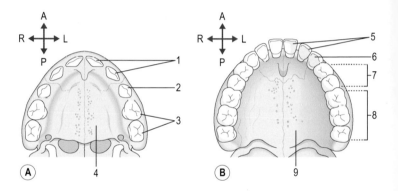

Fig 136 **(A)** The deciduous teeth, seen from below. **(B)** The permanent teeth, seen from below.

1. Incisors
2. Canine
3. Molars
4. Hard palate
5. Incisors
6. Canine
7. Premolars
8. Molars
9. Hard palate

Comments

Anatomical: Humans have two generations of teeth, the temporary deciduous teeth (the milk teeth) and the permanent teeth. Both sets of teeth are present at birth but are immature and lie buried in the mandible and the maxilla. Their periods of eruption start at 6 months and are over by 2 years of age. From the 6th year of life, the deciduous teeth start falling out and are replaced by the permanent teeth. There are 20 deciduous teeth, 10 in the lower jaw and 10 in the upper jaw; these will be replaced by 32 permanent teeth (16 in each jaw). Thus, the permanent dentition consists of 32 teeth and is completed by 21 years of age. There are various tooth types, including the incisor, the canine, the premolar and the molar. During deciduous dentition, both lower and upper jaws each contain two canines, four incisors and four molars. With permanent dentition, the lower and upper jaws each contain two canines, four incisors, four premolars and six molars.

Physiological: The teeth have different functions. The incisors and the canines cut and bite into the food, whereas the premolars and the molars crush and chew the food. Thus, depending on their strength, the teeth cut down the size of the mouthful of food and mix it to form a bolus for swallowing.

Clinical: The signs and symptoms suggestive of dental eruption in the child include excessive salivation, irritability, loss of appetite for solid foods, a rash, diarrhoea, a runny nose, sleep problems and a rise in body temperature.

Section of a tooth

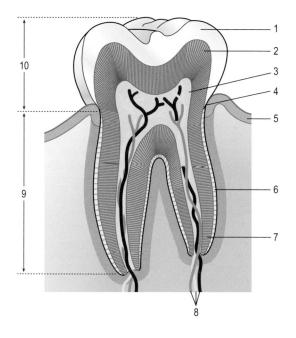

Fig 137

1. Enamel
2. Dentine
3. Pulp chamber
4. Neck
5. Gum
6. Cementum
7. Dentine
8. Blood vessels and nerves
9. Root
10. Crown

Comments

Anatomical: Every tooth is made up of the following structures:

1. The crown, projecting from the roof
2. The root, anchored and held inside its osseous socket and the alveolar bone by cementum, which is a bone-like substance
3. The neck, lying between the crown and the root

The root is implanted into the alveolar bone by one to three prongs. Inside the tooth, the root canal contains blood vessels, lymphatics and nerve fibres that come in via a small apical foramen. The pulp chamber is covered by dentine and enamel, which are hard tissues. The hard enamel coats the dentine and the crown, whereas the cementum coats the root.

Physiological: A tooth is essentially made up of dentine, which is a mineralised tissue, pierced by microtubules containing cytoplasmic processes of the odontoblasts. These cells line the pulp chamber and slowly synthesise dentine throughout life. They also produce new dentine as a reaction to dental caries.

Clinical: Dental caries can be asymptomatic as long as it is confined to the enamel, but later it gives rise to sensitivity or pain in the tooth, which increases with time and becomes an acute pain on eating, drinking a hot or cold beverage and biting.

The salivary glands

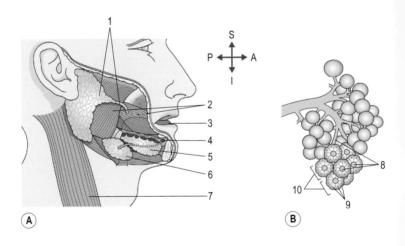

Fig 138 **(A)** Location of the salivary glands. **(B)** Part of a gland, enlarged.

1. Parotid gland and its duct
2. Muscles of the cheek
3. Tongue
4. Opening of the submandibular duct
5. Sublingual gland
6. Submandibular gland
7. Sternocleidomastoid muscle
8. Ductules
9. Secretory sells
10. Acinus

Comments

Anatomical: The salivary glands consist of three pairs of glands located on either side of the face (the parotid and sublingual glands) and in the floor of the mouth (the submandibular glands). They are made up of acini lined by secretory cells. They secrete into ductules that fuse to form ducts, which drain into the mouth.

Physiological: The secretion of saliva ($\approx$1.5 L/day) is controlled by the autonomic nervous system, either by a direct reflex when food enters the mouth or by a conditioned reflex induced by the sight or smell of food.

Clinical: Saliva has many functions, including lubrication of the mouth and the food ingested, tasting, chemical digestion of polysaccharides, and local defence. The signs and symptoms of sialadenitis, with or without sialolithiasis or infections of the floor of the mouth or submandibular region, include the following: pain, a hard swelling, inflammation (redness, heat, pain and swelling), the presence of pus, difficulty in speaking or swallowing and possibly fever.

The oesophagus and some adjacent structures

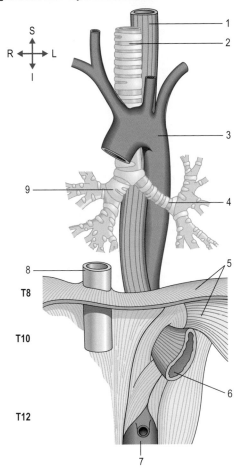

Fig 139

1. Oesophagus
2. Trachea
3. Aorta
4. Left bronchus
5. Diaphragm
6. Lower oesophageal sphincter
7. Aorta
8. Inferior vena cava
9. Right bronchus

Comments

Anatomical: The oesophagus lies in the thorax behind the trachea and the heart and is about 25 cm long. It is a continuation of the pharynx and pierces the diaphragm before joining the stomach. It has a sphincter at each end — the upper oesophageal sphincter at the upper end and the lower oesophageal sphincter at the lower end.

Physiological: The angle formed between the oesophagus and the stomach prevents regurgitation of gastric contents into the oesophagus. It is supplied by the oesophageal, phrenic, gastric and coeliac arteries and is drained by the left gastric, the azygos and the hemiazygos veins.

Clinical: The signs and symptoms of gastrooesophageal reflux include a retrosternal ascending burning sensation on lying down or bending forward, epigastric pain, acid regurgitation, bad breath or halitosis. Painful swallowing and a burning feeling on swallowing are suggestive of oesophagitis.

The muscles of mastication

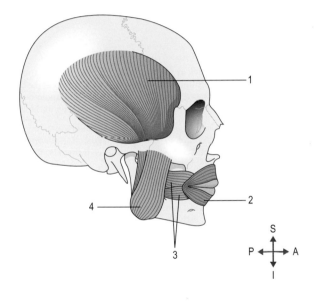

S
P ← → A
I

Fig 140

1. Temporalis muscle
2. Orbicularis oris muscle
3. Buccinator muscle
4. Masseter muscle

Comments

Anatomical: The muscles of mastication are of two types, levators and depressors, and are arranged in pairs symmetrically on both sides of the jaw. The masseter is a muscle made up of two bundles, which arise above from the zygomatic arch and are inserted below, into the angle of the mandible. The temporalis is made up of three bundles, which arise above from the floor of the temporal fossa and are inserted below into the coronoid process of the mandible. The buccinator arises above from the maxilla and is inserted below into the mandible. The orbicularis oris consists of four muscle bundles arranged around the mouth that provide the framework of the lips.

Physiological: The cheek muscles — the masseter, the temporalis, the orbicularis oris and the buccinator — take part in the mastication of food in the mouth. They act along with the teeth, the tongue and the saliva to form a bolus of food for swallowing and to allow the passage of this bolus into the pharynx. The depressor muscles open the mouth by depressing the mandible. The masseter and the temporalis are levators and close the mouth by raising the mandible to contact the maxilla. The levators are more numerous and stronger and work harder than the depressors, which do not need to exert as much force. Gravity brings down the mandible when the muscles are relaxed. The anterior fibres of the temporalis act as a levator; the posterior fibres cause the mandible to recede. The orbicularis oris closes the mouth, allows food to be taken up by suction and controls facial expressions. The buccinator, innervated by the facial nerve, empties the mouth of its contents. The consistency of the food has an influence on the time it spends in the mouth; some foods take longer to be masticated before being swallowed.

Clinical: The force exerted in closing the jaw is reckoned to be equivalent to that exerted by the weight of the subject. Trismus is a continuous and involuntary contraction of the jaw muscles, seen in cases of tetanus and rabies, but also in cases of temporomaxillary arthritis, cellulitis of dental origin and pharyngitis complicated by a tonsillar abscess.

Section of the face and neck showing the location of the structures during swallowing

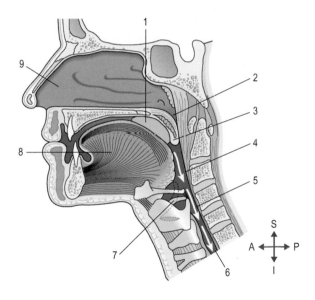

Fig 141

1. Bolus of food on the tongue
2. Nasopharynx
3. Soft palate
4. Oropharynx
5. Laryngopharynx
6. Oesophagus
7. Epiglottis closing the opening of the larynx
8. Tongue
9. Nasal cavity

Comments

Physiological: In addition to supporting the head and allowing it to move, the neck also plays a role in eating, breathing and phonation. Swallowing, whether voluntary or not, occurs in three phases after the bolus of food is formed. The oral phase is due to the voluntary contraction of the muscles of the tongue and the cheeks to move the bolus into the pharynx. The involuntary pharyngeal phase relies on the cumulative actions of the oropharynx, the soft palate, the nasopharynx and the epiglottis to ensure passage of the bolus into the oesophagus, without any risk of reflux towards the mouth or the trachea. The oesophageal phase relies on the lubricating action of mucus on the oesophageal mucosa, peristalsis and the opening of the lower oesophageal sphincter to push the bolus into the stomach.

Clinical: The signs and symptoms of disorders of swallowing include difficulty in masticating or controlling the passage of food or liquids in the mouth, cough, a feeling of suffocation as food or liquids spill into the respiratory tract or the throat and pain on swallowing.

The stomach and adjacent structures

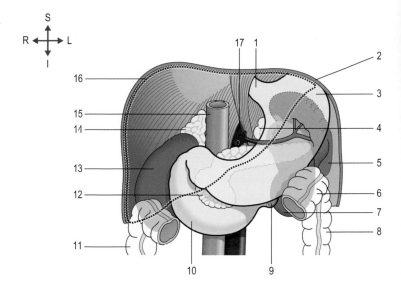

Fig 142

1. Oesophagus
2. Diaphragm (showing the edge of a cross section)
3. Stomach
4. Left suprarenal gland
5. Spleen
6. Transverse colon (transected)
7. Left kidney
8. Descending colon
9. First part of duodenum
10. Duodenum
11. Ascending colon
12. Head of pancreas
13. Right kidney
14. Right suprarenal gland
15. Inferior vena cava
16. Edge of liver (shown as *dotted line*)
17. Abdominal aorta

Comments

Anatomical: The stomach is related to many structures as it lies in the epigastrium, the umbilical region and the left hypochondrium. These include the following:

1. To the right, the liver and the duodenum
2. To the left, the diaphragm and the spleen
3. Posteriorly, the pancreas, the spleen, the right and left suprarenal glands and the abdominal aorta
4. Superiorly, the diaphragm, the oesophagus and the left lobe of the liver
5. Inferiorly, the small intestine and the transverse colon
6. Anteriorly, the left lobe of the liver and the abdominal wall

It is about 15 cm in height, and its capacity ranges from 0.5 to 4 litres.

Physiological: The stomach receives food chewed in the mouth and swallowed into the oesophagus. It mixes the food and stores it for some time to allow the digestive enzymes (pepsins) to break down the proteins into polypeptides. The gastric contents are transformed into chyme by the gastric juices. The acidity of the stomach provides a nonspecific type of protection against microbes and, by making iron salts soluble, it promotes iron absorption by the small intestine.

Clinical: The anatomical location of the stomach explains why gastric pain can be localised or can spread to other parts of the body. A gastric ulcer can be associated with a localised cramp-like epigastric pain or with a painful sensation of hunger, which is relieved by taking food or antacids and is rhythmically related to meals, with a period of relief lasting about 2 hours. It can sometimes give rise to a feeling of discomfort unrelated to meals. The pain can also occur in the right, left or posterior hypochondrium. Haemorrhage can be a complication of a gastric ulcer.

Longitudinal section of the stomach

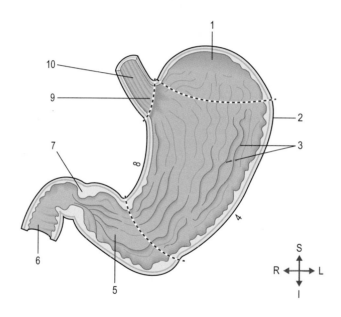

Fig 143

1. Fundus
2. Body
3. Folds
4. Greater curvature
5. Pylorus
6. Duodenum
7. Pyloric sphincter
8. Lesser curvature
9. Lower oesophageal sphincter
10. Oesophagus

Comments

Anatomical: The stomach has two curvatures, the J-shaped lesser curvature on its right medial aspect and the greater curvature on its left lateral aspect. It consists of three parts — the fundus, the body and the pylorus. It is linked to the oesophagus by the lower oesophageal sphincter and, at its distal end, it passes into the duodenum via the pyloric sphincter.

Physiological: During digestion, the stomach plays a mechanical and a secretory role. The lower oesophageal sphincter, which is normally closed, and the cardiac incisura at the oesophagogastric junction normally prevent acid reflux upstream. The pyloric sphincter is relaxed and open or closed, depending on whether stomach is relatively inactive or active; it allows the passage of the bolus of food into the duodenum. It is closed when the bolus presents itself and opens to allow it to enter the duodenum. The pylorus is a muscular part of the stomach that ensures adequate digestion of the bolus of food in the stomach and restricts the passage of large food particles into the small intestine. Coming after the pylorus, the duodenum is the first segment of the small intestine.

Clinical: The rate at which the stomach empties varies according to the type of food ingested. The time it takes to empty increases progressively, depending on whether the meal is rich in carbohydrates, proteins or fat. Vomiting after a meal suggests the presence of a stenotic lesion, and it can also be related to the ingestion of gastric irritants, microbial or chemical.

The muscular coat of the stomach wall

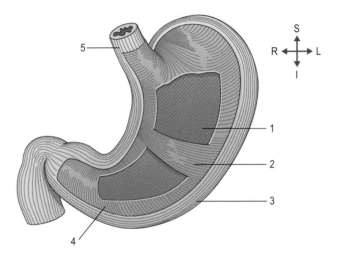

Fig 144 The cuts have been removed to show the three layers.

1. Internal oblique muscle layer
2. Middle circular muscle layer
3. Outer longitudinal muscle layer
4. Middle circular fibres
5. Oesophagus

Comments

Anatomical: The stomach also contains the basic four-layered structure of the alimentary tract. Its muscular coat consists of three layers of smooth muscle—longitudinal, circular and oblique—unlike the other digestive organs, with only two layers. The circular muscle wall is at its strongest between the pylorus and the pyloric sphincter.

Physiological: Those three smooth muscle coats are responsible for the essential and characteristic mixing and peristaltic activity of the stomach. They allow the food to be broken up mechanically, be exposed to the pepsins and the gastric juices and form chyme for transfer to the duodenum. The mucosa contains longitudinal folds that become stretched as the stomach fills. Gastric motility and secretory activity are enhanced by stimulation of the parasympathetic system. The stomach is richly supplied and drained by the right and left gastric and gastroepiploic arteries and veins. These arteries are branches of the coeliac artery, and the veins drain into the superior mesenteric vein.

Clinical: Because of its rich blood supply, haemorrhage is a frequent complication of an ulcer or a cancer associated with erosion of the superficial vessels. An upper gastrointestinal haemorrhage presents as haematemesis (vomiting of blood) or as melaena (dark stools with altered blood). Tiredness can be due to anaemia. Anxiety and stress can trigger digestive symptoms such as loss of appetite, nausea, heartburn, belching and a bloated feeling. Eating the wrong foods (e.g., fatty, sweet or spicy foods), drinking fizzy drinks or alcohol and eating too much cause gastrointestinal discomfort by slowing down digestion. The bloating is due to the build up of gas in the intestines and reflects a slowing down of intestinal peristalsis.

The microstructure of the gastric mucosa, showing the gastric glands

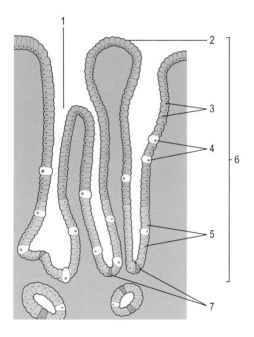

Fig 145

1. Gastric crypt
2. Surface epithelium
3. Mucous neck cells
4. Parietal cells
5. Chief cells
6. Gastric glands
7. Neuroendocrine cells

Comments

Anatomical: The gastric mucosa folds or unfolds, depending on whether the stomach, which varies in volume, is active or not. It contains a vast number of gastric glands located under its surface, into which they open.

Physiological: The production of gastric juices is triggered by the smell or the sight of food, by its entry into the stomach and by hormones. Gastric glands secrete about 2 litres of gastric juice, which mixes progressively with the bolus of food to increase its acidity, break it up and liquefy it. The chyme is then ready to be propelled into the duodenum. In addition to the enzymes that break down the food into simple molecules, the gastric juices contain many substances such as water, mineral salts, hydrochloric acid, mucus, enzymes (pepsinogens) and proteins. Some of the glands secrete mucus, which protects the stomach wall against the acidic environment. The gastric secretions kill some bacteria. Gastric secretion is enhanced by stimulation of the parasympathetic nervous system and reduced by stimulation of the sympathetic nervous system. Contractions of the stomach blend the food, mixing it with the gastric juices.

Clinical: Dyspepsia (indigestion) is a feeling of heaviness, being too full, bloating associated with belching and pain occurring during or after meals. Belching following a meal is due to the ingestion of air during eating and its expulsion from the upper part of the stomach. Heartburn and retrosternal pain are symptomatic of gastrooesophageal reflux or gastritis (inflammation of the stomach). Excess acid causes erosion of the stomach lining, leading to ulceration, with or without associated haemorrhage. Nausea, vomiting and diarrhoea are symptoms of gastroenteritis (inflammation of the gastrointestinal tract) or food poisoning.

The duodenum and adjacent structures

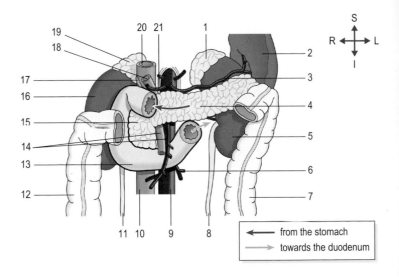

from the stomach
towards the duodenum

Fig 146

1. Left suprarenal gland
2. Spleen
3. Splenic artery
4. Body of pancreas
5. Left kidney
6. Inferior mesenteric artery
7. Descending colon
8. Left ureter
9. Aorta
10. Superior vena cava
11. Right ureter

12. Ascending colon
13. Duodenum
14. Superior mesenteric artery and vein
15. Head of pancreas
16. Right kidney
17. Common bile duct
18. Portal vein
19. Right suprarenal gland
20. Inferior vena cava
21. Hepatic artery

Comments

Anatomical: The duodenum, which is stuck to the peritoneum, is the first of the three segments of the small intestine, the other two being the jejunum and the ileum. It is the fixed segment that follows the pylorus of the stomach and is followed by the jejunum at the duodenojejunal angle. Located in the abdomen and measuring about 25 cm in length, it is related to the head and the neck of the pancreas, the liver, the common bile duct, the colon, the portal vein, and the superior mesenteric vessels (artery and vein). Its wall consists of four tissue layers. Its mucosa has folds, villi and intestinal glands that secrete digestive enzymes.

Physiological: The duodenum participates in digestion without continuous peristaltic activity. Its mucosa contains intestinal glands that secrete the digestive enzymes. Its endocrine cells secrete secretin and cholecystokinin, which control the secretion of pancreatic juice by the exocrine pancreas, the release of bile from the gall bladder, and the passage of the pancreatic juice and bile into the duodenum as a result of relaxation of the sphincter of Oddi. The chyme is then mixed with the enzymes, intestinal secretions and bile, leading to further digestion of proteins, carbohydrates and lipids.

Clinical: In coeliac disease, due to a genuine gluten intolerance, the duodenal papillae become atrophic, leading to signs and symptoms of malabsorption — chronic diarrhoea, loss of weight and multiple nutritional deficiencies, especially of iron, folate and vitamin B_{12}.

The jejunum, the ileum and adjacent structures

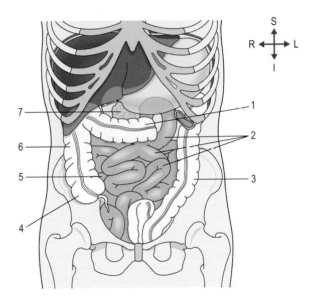

Fig 147

1. Transverse colon
2. Jejunum and ileum
3. Descending colon
4. Caecum
5. Terminal part of the ileum
6. Ascending colon
7. Pancreas

Comments

Anatomical: The jejunum, measuring about 2 m long, and the ileum, about 3 m long, are the middle and distal segments of the small bowel, respectively. The ileum contains the ileocaecal valve.

Physiological: Both the jejunum and the ileum play a role in digestion. They have propulsive and secretory functions, with the production of intestinal juices and hormones. They contribute to the production of intestinal juices, which amount to almost 1500 mL per day. At the distal end of the ileum, the proteins, carbohydrates and lipids have all been broken down, respectively, into amino acids, monosaccharides and fatty acids and monoglycerides. The ileocaecal valve prevents the reflux of caecal contents into the ileum.

Clinical: The signs and symptoms of Crohn's disease, a chronic inflammatory process involving the digestive tract, include abdominal pain in the right iliac fossa, alternating bouts of diarrhoea and constipation, watery, blood-free stools, weight loss and low-grade fever. It is a chronic inflammatory disease of the alimentary tract associated with erosions or ulcerations, occasionally involving the stomach and the duodenum. There can also be extraintestinal involvement of the joints, the skin and the eyes.

The intestinal villi

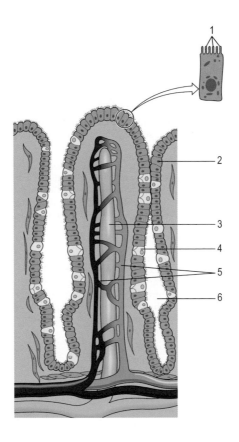

Fig 148

1. Microvilli
2. Enterocyte
3. Lacteal
4. Goblet cell
5. Capillary network
6. Intestinal crypt

Comments

Anatomical: The villi are tiny, finger-like projections of the intestinal mucosa that are 0.5 to 1 mm long. They consist of cylindrical epithelial cells or enterocytes covered with microvilli and contain a capillary and lymphatic network. Among the enterocytes lie the mucus-secreting goblet cells. The tubular intestinal glands (crypts of Lieberkühn) lie between the villi.

Physiological: The enterocytes play a role in digestion. The mucosal epithelium is replaced approximately every 4 days. The epithelial cells synthesise digestive enzymes that coat the microvilli, where they mix with the intestinal juices and complete the digestion of carbohydrates, proteins and lipids. These digestive end products are absorbed and enter the blood capillaries and the lymphatics. Fat absorption imparts a milky appearance to the lymph — hence, the name of chyliferous lacteals for the lymphatic capillaries.

Clinical: Atrophy of the villi causing malabsorption of nutrients can occur in many diseases, with the most common being coeliac disease. Other causes include antibiotic and anticancer drugs, parasites, immunodeficiency and radiotherapy.

Nutrient absorption by the intestinal villi

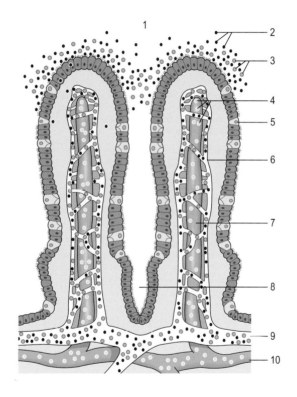

Fig 149

1. Intestinal lumen
2. Carbohydrates
3. Polypeptides
4. Lipid molecules
5. Goblet cell
6. Blood capillary
7. Central lacteal
8. Intestinal crypt
9. Blood in the capillaries
10. Fatty contents of the lacteals

Comments

Anatomical: The circular folds of the mucosal membrane contain numerous villi.

Physiological: The enterocytes play a role in the chemical digestion of food. The intestinal crypts that secrete the intestinal juices are stimulated mechanically by the chyme with the help of secretin. The enzymes — peptidases, lipase, saccharase, maltase and lactase — break down the proteins into amino acids, the carbohydrates into monosaccharides and the lipids into fatty acids and monoglycerides. The peptidases, secreted by the pancreas, are activated by enterokinase, which is secreted by the duodenum. Two modes of absorption, osmosis and diffusion, allow the digestive end products to enter the blood capillaries and the lymphatics. Because absorption of fats imparts a milky appearance to the lymph, these lymphatics are called chyliferous lacteals. Water and water-soluble vitamins cross the cell membranes by osmosis. The monosaccharides enter by diffusion to reach the villous capillaries. The lipid-soluble substances, like the vitamins, the fatty acids and the monoglycerides, diffuse into the chyliferous lacteals.

Clinical: The signs and symptoms of coeliac disease include tiredness, abdominal pains, diarrhoea with fatty stools, weight loss, malnutrition, growth retardation in the child, joint pains, oedema of the lower limbs and infertility. Its accurate clinical diagnosis is vital and requires histological proof following biopsy via a fibrescope of the duodenal mucosa.

Mean volumes of fluid ingested, secreted, absorbed and excreted daily by the alimentary tract

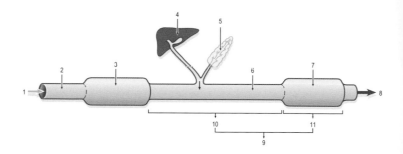

Fig 150

1. Water (1200 mL)
2. Saliva (1500 mL)
3. Gastric juice (2000 mL)
4. Bile (200 mL)
5. Pancreatic juice (1500 mL)
0. Intestinal juice (1500 mL)

7. Colon
8. Stools (100 mL)
9. Absorbed into the bloodstream
10. 6700 mL
11. 1400 ml

Comments

Physiological: A large amount of fluid enters the alimentary tract daily. Only 1500 mL is absorbed by the small intestine, and the rest passes into the large intestine. The water from drinks is easily absorbed by diffusion across the intestinal membrane. The secretion along the alimentary tract of saliva, gastric juice, pancreatic juice, intestinal juice and bile cooperates to ensure the digestion of proteins, lipids and carbohydrates. The substances left undigested are eliminated in the stools at the distal end of the tract, the rectum.

Clinical: The composition, consistency, colour and volume of the stools vary according to the amount of water ingested, the diet and the digestive process. These stools, weighing between 150 and 200 g daily, are the residues of the digestion of food after its passage through the digestive tract. They consist of undigested foods such as cellulose, intestinal epithelial cells that are constantly being replaced and bacteria from to the intestinal flora. The colour of the stools, due to the presence of stercobilin (a metabolic product of bilirubin), varies from beige to brown, depending on the foods ingested. Beetroot or spinach alters the colour to red or green. Normal stools, made up of 75% water and 25% dry matter, are semisolid and coated with mucus, but can vary in consistency. Diarrhoea is associated with a higher percentage of water and a total stool weight in excess of 200 g daily. The length of the gut helps reduce the amount of water in stools. Examining the stools allows one to evaluate the function of the digestive tract. Steatorrhoea, due to the presence of fat in the stools, suggests some form of deficiency in the digestive process. Constipation, diarrhoea and pain suggest some problem with intestinal transit. The presence of red or dark blood raises the possibility of haemorrhage, an ulcer or even cancer. The first stools passed by a newborn, called meconium, are dark green and characteristic.

The segments of the large intestine and their locations

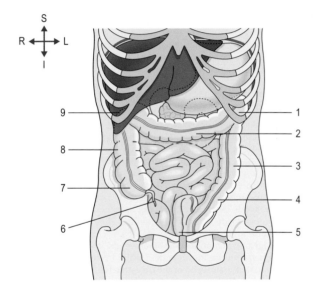

Fig 151

1. Left (splenic) colic flexure
2. Transverse colon
3. Descending colon
4. Sigmoid colon
5. Rectum
6. Vermiform appendix
7. Caecum
8. Ascending colon
9. Right (hepatic) colic flexure

Comments

Anatomical: The four basic tissue layers of the gastrointestinal tract are also present in the colon. The large intestine is about 1.5 m in length and 6.5 cm in diameter. It consists of the caecum, the ascending colon, the transverse colon, the descending colon, the sigmoid colon and the rectum. The vermiform appendix is a slender tubular structure measuring about 8 cm in length that arises from the caecum.

Physiological: The large intestine plays a role in the absorption of water, mineral salts and vitamins, in the microbial synthesis of vitamin K and folic acid and in the peristaltic evacuation of semisolid stools.

Clinical: Chronic diarrhoea, bloodstained or slimy, and associated with haemorrhage during severe painful exacerbations, rectal pain (tenesmus), colic, fatigue and loss of weight are symptoms of ulcerative colitis, characterised by episodes of severe inflammatory damage to the colonic mucosa.

The interior of the caecum

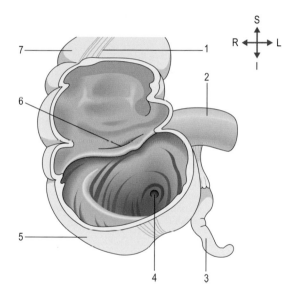

Fig 152

1. Taenia coli
2. Terminal ileum
3. Vermiform appendix
4. Orifice of the vermiform appendix
5. Caecum
6. Ileocaecal valve
7. Ascending colon

Comments

Anatomical: The dilated pouch-like caecum is the first part of the large intestine and is continuous with the ascending colon. It has a different arrangement of its longitudinal muscle fibres, which are gathered into separate bundles (taeniae) instead of forming a continuous sheet. The shorter taeniae on the surface of the caecum give it the appearance of a puckered pouch. The ileocaecal valve prevents reflux into the ileum. The vermiform appendix is a slender tubular structure measuring about 8 cm in length; it arises from the caecum and ends blindly distally. It contains all the basic structures of the digestive tract, except for a larger amount of lymphoid tissue.

Physiological: The appendix has no digestive function.

Clinical: The signs and symptoms of acute appendicitis are pain in the right iliac fossa, spreading to the lumbar region and the root of the right thigh, and associated with nausea and vomiting, constipation and fever. Abdominal pain, often severe, associated with failure to pass stools and flatus, and with gaseous abdominal distention, is suggestive of intestinal obstruction. The signs and symptoms of Crohn's disease are rectal bleeding associated with abdominal pain in the right iliac fossa, alternating bouts of diarrhoea and constipation, loss of weight and low-grade fever.

Arrangement of the muscle fibres of the colon, rectum and anus

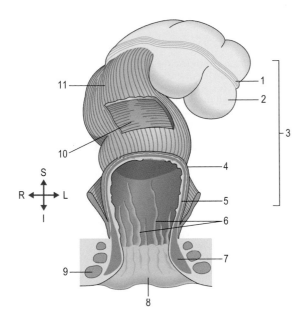

Fig 153 The cut portions have been removed to show the muscle layers.

1. Taenia coli
2. Sigmoid colon
3. Rectum
4. Longitudinal fibres
5. Circular fibres
6. Anal columns
7. Internal anal sphincter (smooth muscle)
8. Anus
9. External anal sphincter (striated muscle)
10. Circular fibres (after removal of the longitudinal fibres)
11. Longitudinal fibres forming a continuous sheet

Comments

Anatomical: The four basic layers of the gastrointestinal tract are present in the colon, rectum and anus, but the arrangement of the longitudinal muscle fibres is different in the colon, where they are gathered into separate bundles (taeniae coli) as far down as the rectosigmoid junction.

Physiological: The colon is still an active part of the alimentary tract, with mucus-secreting goblet cells present. Defaecation is controlled by sphincters. The internal anal sphincter is controlled by the autonomic nervous system, whereas contraction of the external anal sphincter is under voluntary control.

Clinical: The signs and symptoms of anal fissure include a burning pain of variable intensity on defaecation, pruritus ani, spasms of the external sphincter and traces of blood in the stools. This picture is made worse by constipation associated with pain on defaecation. Disturbances in intestinal mobility, such as constipation, diarrhoea or alternating episodes of diarrhoea and constipation, with blood in the stool, bouts of colicky abdominal pain, unexplained weight loss and low-grade fever are suggestive of a polyp or of a cancer. However, cancer can be asymptomatic for a long time. Bright red blood in the stools most often indicates the presence of haemorrhoids.

The pancreas in relation to the duodenum and the biliary tract

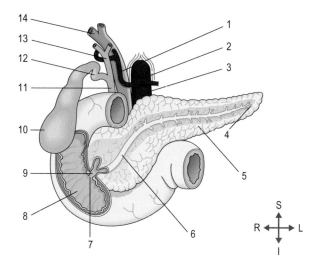

Fig 154 Part of the anterior wall of the duodenum has been excised.

1. Hepatic artery
2. Coeliac artery
3. Aorta
4. Tail of pancreas
5. Body of pancreas
6. Pancreatic duct
7. Duodenal papilla
8. Interior of duodenum
9. Hepatopancreatic ampulla
10. Gall bladder
11. Common bile duct
12. Cystic duct
13. Hepatic duct
14. Portal vein

Comments

Anatomical: The pancreas, which is about 13 cm long, is a mixed endocrine and exocrine gland lying in the epigastrium and the left hypochondrium. It consists of a head, a body and a tail. It is related anatomically to the stomach, the duodenum, the kidney, the spleen, the abdominal aorta and the inferior vena cava. It is made up of the islets of Langerhans and lobules of acini lined by secretory cells. It is supplied by the splenic and superior mesenteric arteries. The splenic and the mesenteric veins, along with their tributaries, join to form the portal vein.

Physiological: The pancreas secretes insulin and glucagon, two hormones that enter the blood directly and are responsible for the control of blood glucose levels. The acini secrete the pancreatic juices, which are transported by the pancreatic duct, and its enzymes help digest proteins, carbohydrates and fats.

Clinical: The signs and symptoms of diabetes include hyperglycaemia, ketosis, ketoacidosis, glycosuria, polyuria and weight loss, which are related to pancreatic endocrine insufficiency. The signs and symptoms of an acute or chronic pancreatitis include acute epigastric pain, with or without spread into the back and/or the left hypochondrium; it is of slowly progressive or rapid onset and is eased by sitting up in bed or turning onto the left side. To relieve the pain, the patient adopts the curled-up position. Additional complications include nausea, vomiting and abdominal distention and, more alarmingly, tachycardia and hypotension.

The liver (1)

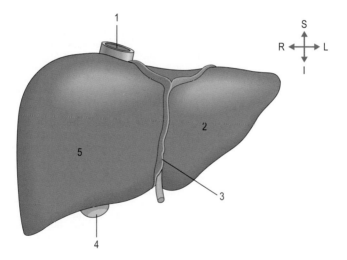

Fig 155 Anterior view.

1. Superior vena cava
2. Left lobe
3. Falciform ligament
4. Gall bladder
5. Right lobe

Comments

Anatomical: The liver is a massive gland located in the epigastrium and the right and left hypochondria. It is divided into two lobes separated by the falciform ligament. The lobes are made of lobules containing the hepatocytes. The shape of the liver allows it to adapt to that of the diaphragm. It is not fully covered by the peritoneum and is related to the gall bladder.

Physiological: The functions of the liver include detoxification, synthesis and storage. The hepatocytes secrete bile. It plays a role in the metabolism of carbohydrates, proteins and lipids, the breakdown of red blood cells, antimicrobial defence, the detoxification of harmful substances and drugs, the inactivation of hormones (e.g., insulin, glucagon, cortisol, aldosterone, thyroid hormones and sex hormones), and heat production.

Clinical. Signs and symptoms of acute hepatitis include nausea, loss of appetite, jaundice observed in the skin and eyes, pale stools, dark urine, itching, fatigue and muscle pains. Jaundice is a yellow or yellowish discolouration of the skin and the conjunctiva resulting from increased levels of bilirubin in the blood. Severe weight loss, loss of appetite, nausea, pain in the upper quadrant of the abdomen and a palpable mass are suggestive of liver cancer, which is often a complication of cirrhosis of the liver.

The liver (2)

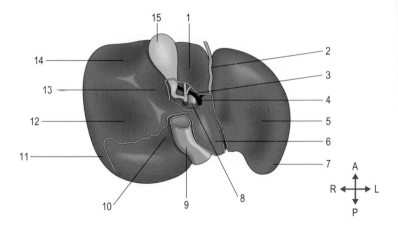

Fig 156 Inferior view (turned up to show the posterior surface).

1. Quadrate lobe
2. Falciform ligament
3. Bile duct
4. Hepatic artery
5. Gastric impression
6. Caudate lobe
7. Left lobe
8. Portal vein
9. Inferior vena cava
10. Right suprarenal impression
11. Right lobe
12. Right renal impression
13. Duodenal impression
14. Colic impression
15. Gall bladder

Comments

Anatomical: The liver is related to these adjacent organs: the diaphragm, the vertebral column, the lower ribs, the anterior abdominal wall, the oesophagus, the stomach, the bile ducts, the gall bladder, the duodenum, the colon, the right kidney and the right suprarenal gland. It is supplied by the hepatic artery and the portal vein.

Physiological: The liver secretes bile (about 750 mL/day), which helps in the digestion of lipids and the excretion of bilirubin. It stores glycogen, inactivates hormones (e.g., insulin, glucagon, cortisol, aldosterone, thyroid hormones and sex hormones), metabolises proteins, carbohydrates and fats and is active in antimicrobial defence, detoxification and heat production.

Clinical: The signs and symptoms of cirrhosis include generalised weakness, weight loss, ascites (the presence of fluid inside the peritoneal cavity) and jaundice (yellowing of the skin and mucous membranes). Ascites is the result of the accumulation of more than 1500 mL of fluid in the peritoneal cavity.

A hepatic lobule

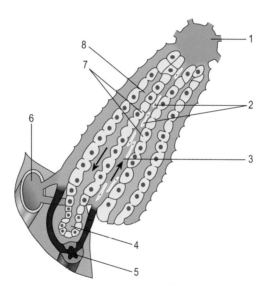

Fig 157 Shown is the direction of the flow of blood and bile in the hepatic lobule.

1. Central vein (tributary of a hepatic vein)
2. Hepatic macrophages (Kupffer cells)
3. Sinusoid full of blood
4. Bile canaliculus
5. Branch of hepatic artery
6. Branch of portal vein
7. Hepatocytes
8. Bile canaliculus

Comments

Anatomical: The hepatic lobes are made of small functional lobules. Each lobule contains lymphatic tissue and a network of lymphatic vessels. These lobules are made up of pairs of cuboidal cells, the hepatocytes, and are arranged in cords radiating away from the central vein. Between these hepatocytes lie the sinusoids, which are blood vessels that are filled with blood coming from the portal vein and the hepatic artery and that drain into the central vein of the lobule. The sinusoids are flanked by macrophages (Kupffer cells). Each cord of hepatocytes has a sinusoid on one side and a bile canaliculus on the other. The bile canaliculi form the intrahepatic bile ducts, which give rise to the right and left hepatic ducts.

Physiological: There is mixing of arterial blood and venous blood along the hepatocytes. The macrophages ingest and destroy aged cells and foreign cells present in the intrahepatic blood. The liver secretes bile, which is drained by the right and left hepatic ducts.

Clinical: Jaundice, a change in the colour of the stools, dark urine, pruritus, fat malabsorption, steatorrhoea and loss of weight are suggestive of a cholestatic syndrome due to malfunction of the intrahepatic or extrahepatic biliary system.

Direction of the flow of bile from liver to duodenum

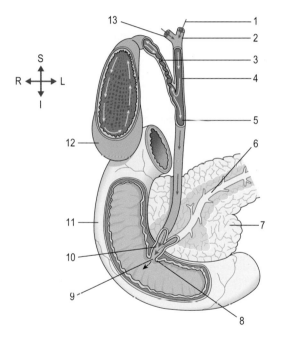

Fig 158

1. Bile coming from the liver
2. Left hepatic duct
3. Cystic duct
4. Common hepatic duct
5. Common bile duct
6. Main pancreatic duct
7. Head of pancreas
8. Hepatopancreatic sphincter (sphincter of Oddi)
9. Major duodenal papilla
10. Hepatopancreatic ampulla
11. Duodenum
12. Gall bladder
13. Right hepatic duct

Comments

Anatomical: The bile secreted by the hepatocytes drains via the right and left hepatic ducts, which fuse to form the common hepatic duct before it joins the cystic duct coming from the gall bladder. These two ducts join to form the common bile duct, which runs behind the head of the pancreas on its way to join the main pancreatic duct, and form the hepatopancreatic ampulla, which in turn opens into the major duodenal papilla at the sphincter of Oddi. The pear-shaped gall bladder is attached to the inferoposterior surface of the liver by connective tissue and is only partly covered by peritoneum. It consists of a dilated fundus, a body and a neck, which is continuous with the cystic duct. The muscular coat of the gall bladder contains an additional oblique layer of smooth muscle. When empty, the mucous membrane is folded. It is supplied by the cystic artery and drained by the cystic vein, which joins the portal vein.

Physiological: The gall bladder stores the bile and releases the stored bile. Bile runs both ways in the cystic duct as it flows into and out of the gall bladder. Contraction of the muscular coat of the gall bladder propels the bile present in the biliary ducts towards the duodenum, and the hepatopancreatic sphincter relaxes. Bile plays a role in the digestion of lipids and the excretion of bilirubin.

Clinical: Cholecystitis, an acute inflammation of the gall bladder, occurs when a gallstone is caught in the cystic duct; it is accompanied by a severe pain in the epigastrium or the right hypochondrium. Potential complications include infection and peritonitis, following rupture of the gall bladder wall.

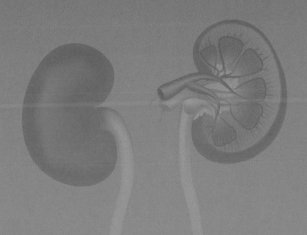

Urinary system

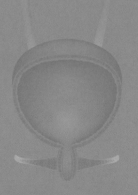

The components of the urinary system (without the urethra) and some adjacent structures

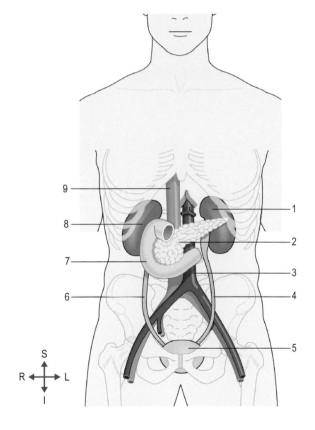

Fig 159

1. Left kidney
2. Pancreas
3. Aorta
4. Left ureter
5. Bladder
6. Right ureter
7. Duodenum
8. Right kidney
9. Inferior vena cava

Comments

Anatomical: The urinary system consists of two kidneys, two ureters, one bladder and one urethra.

Physiological: The urinary system has vital excretory functions, such as the formation of urine to maintain water and electrolyte homoeostasis (water, electrolyte and acid–base balance), the excretion of metabolic waste products (nitrogenous compounds such as urea, creatinine and uric acid, ions in excess of body needs and some drugs), the secretion of erythropoietin (a hormone stimulating the production of red cells), the secretion of renin (an enzyme critical for the control of arterial blood pressure) and the transport and storage of urine.

Clinical: The bladder fills with urine at the rate of about 60 mL per hour. The collection of urine every hour or every 24 hours allows renal function to be monitored. Signs and symptoms suggestive of obstruction in the tract or of renal disease (e.g., renal stones, infections and other lesions) include severe pain in the lumbar region, increase in volume and frequency of urination, oliguria (a urine volume <400 mL in 24 hours), anuria (absence of urine), pyuria (pus in the urine) and haematuria (blood in the urine). There may be other signs, such as oedema and arterial hypertension.

Anterior view of the kidneys, showing their sites of contact with adjacent structures

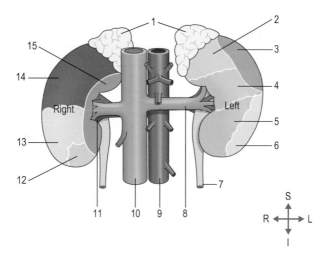

Fig 160

1. Suprarenal glands
2. Stomach
3. Spleen
4. Pancreas
5. Jejunum
6. Left (splenic) colic flexure
7. Ureter
8. Renal vein
9. Aorta
10. Inferior vena cava
11. Renal artery
12. Small intestine
13. Right (hepatic) colic flexure
14. Liver
15. Duodenum

Comments

Anatomical: The bean-shaped kidneys are located on either side of the vertebral column between the 12th thoracic vertebra (T12) and 3rd lumbar vertebra (L3). The renal fascia, made up of connective tissue, surrounds each kidney and keeps it tethered in contact with the adjacent organs. The relations of the right kidney include the right suprarenal gland, the right lobe of the liver, the duodenum and the right colic flexure of the colon. Both kidneys are in contact with the diaphragm and the muscles of the posterior abdominal wall. The relations of the left kidney include the left suprarenal gland, the spleen, the stomach, the pancreas, the jejunum and the left colic flexure. The blood supply of the kidney depends on the renal artery and the renal vein, which enter or leave at the renal hilum.

Clinical: Chronic renal failure is very often associated with a reduction in the size of the kidneys. Signs and symptoms of renal cancer may include lumbar pain, haematuria, weight loss and fever. It can also be detected by chance during an ultrasound or a computed tomography scan performed for some other reason.

Longitudinal section of the right kidney

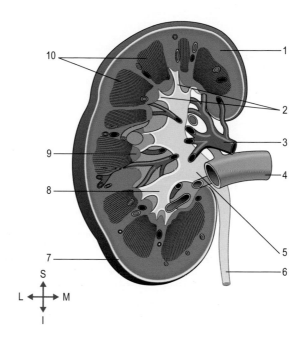

Fig 161

1. Cortex
2. Minor calyces
3. Renal artery
4. Renal vein
5. Renal pelvis
6. Ureter
7. Capsule
8. Major calyx
9. Renal papilla
10. Medulla (pyramids)

Comments

Anatomical: The kidney consists of three tissue layers. On the outside, there is a fibrous capsule that surrounds it and overlies the cortex, which is a layer of brown tissue sandwiched between the capsule and the pyramids. The medulla, the innermost layer of the kidney, consists of the renal pyramids, which appear striated because of the presence of the collecting ducts as they carry urine to the calyces. The blood vessels, the nerves and the ureter pass through the hilum, which forms a concave border in the middle of the medial aspect of the kidney.

Physiological: The urine formed in the nephron is moved along by intratubular hydrostatic pressure. It passes through a renal papilla at the apex of a pyramid, drains into the calyces and the renal pelvis and enters the bladder, where it is stored until it is excreted.

Clinical: The presence of small renal stones (nephrolithiasis) in the calyces can lead to renal colic if the stones become impacted in the ureter and can cause very severe acute pain in the lumbar region, radiating towards the external genitalia. The stones are formed when some normally dissolved urinary constituents precipitate as a result of some metabolic disease, dehydration or a change in the urinary pH during some infections.

A nephron and its associated blood vessels

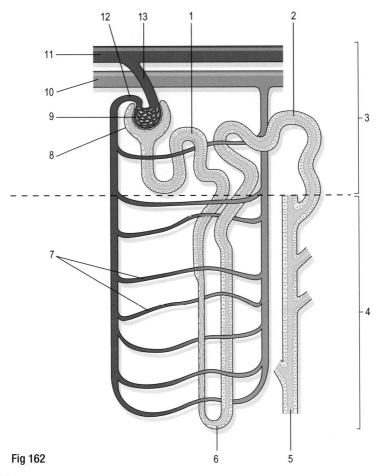

Fig 162

1. Proximal convoluted tubule
2. Distal convoluted tubule
3. Renal cortex
4. Renal medulla
5. Collecting duct
6. Loop of Henle
7. Peritubular capillaries
8. Glomerular capsule
9. Glomerulus
10. Tributary of renal vein
11. Branch of renal artery
12. Efferent arteriole
13. Afferent arteriole

Comments

Anatomical: Each kidney may contain up to 1.5 million functional units, called *nephrons*. Each nephron is made up of a glomerular capsule (Bowman's capsule), a proximal convoluted tubule, a loop of Henle and a distal convoluted tubule leading to a collecting duct. The nephron lies in the renal cortex and in the renal medulla. The blood vessels are innervated by fibres of the sympathetic and parasympathetic systems. The renal artery enters via the hilum and then divides into smaller arteries to form the arterioles. An afferent arteriole enters the glomerular capsule and divides into small capillaries, forming the glomerulus, from which the efferent arterioles arise.

Physiological: Urine formation depends on three processes—simple filtration, selective reabsorption and secretion. The filtration of water and small molecules takes place across the semipermeable membranes of the glomerular capillaries and the glomerular capsule as a result of the pressure difference between the osmotic pressure of blood and the hydrostatic pressure of the filtrate. The blood cells, plasma proteins and large molecules are not filtered. The glomerular filtrate has roughly the same composition as blood plasma. The filtrate is reabsorbed passively or actively into the blood in the proximal convoluted tubule. The substances reabsorbed include sodium, potassium, chloride, calcium, phosphate, glucose and amino acids. This reabsorption has a threshold, depending on whether or not the organism needs it, and is controlled by certain hormones. The reabsorption of nitrogenous waste products is limited. Secretion of hydrogen ions is important for the maintenance of homoeostasis.

The serial arrangement of the blood vessels in the kidney

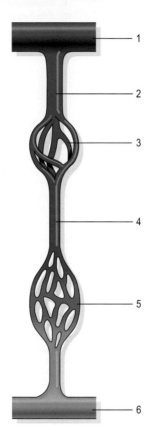

Fig 163

1. Renal artery
2. Afferent arteriole
3. Glomerulus
4. Efferent arteriole
5. Peritubular capillaries (supplying the nephron)
6. Renal vein

Comments

Anatomical: The kidney is a very vascular organ. The renal artery divides sequentially into segmental, interlobar, arcuate and interlobular arteries before giving rise to the arterioles. The afferent arteriole enters the glomerular capsule and then divides further into small capillaries to form the glomerulus. An efferent arteriole exits the capsule to give rise to the interlobular veins and the interlobar veins, which drain into the renal vein, as it leaves the renal hilum to join the inferior vena cava.

Physiological: The renal artery supplies the kidney with blood. The difference in the diameters of the afferent and efferent arterioles — and hence the difference in their intraluminal pressure — allows filtration to occur. This process does not allow large molecules such as plasma proteins and blood cells to be filtered.

Clinical: Haematuria is a common clinical finding in diseases of the kidneys because of their rich vascularity. The risk of haemorrhage is higher in cases of rupture or trauma to the kidney. Gross haematuria, lumbar pain and clinical signs of shock (e.g., tachycardia, arterial hypotension) are suggestive of renal trauma. Haematuria, a sudden acute and intense pain in the flank or in the abdomen, described as a stabbing pain, nausea, vomiting and a feeling of sickness are the signs and symptoms of renal infarction.

Glomerular filtration

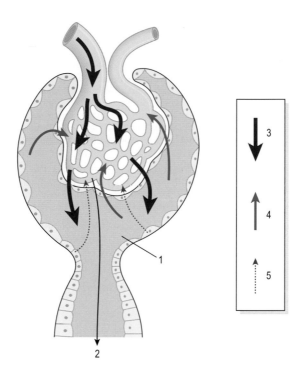

Fig 164

1. Glomerular capsule
2. Net filtration pressure (1.3 kPa, or 10 mmHg)
3. Glomerular hydrostatic pressure (7.3 kPa, or 60 mmHg)
4. Glomerular osmotic pressure (4 kPa, or 32 mmHg)
5. Glomerular hydrostatic pressure (2 kPa, or 18 mmHg)

Comments

Anatomical: At the upper end of the nephron, the cup-shaped glomerular capsule or Bowman's capsule surrounds the glomerulus, which is a network of arterial capillaries.

Physiological: Filtration occurs across the semipermeable membrane of the glomerular capillaries and the glomerular capsule as a result of the pressure difference between the osmotic pressure of the blood and the hydrostatic pressure of the filtrate.

Clinical: Haematuria and proteinuria are the two main signs of glomerular disease. Oedema and arterial hypertension may also be present, indicating renal insufficiency. The predominance of one of these findings, along with a significant proteinuria and a variable rate of progression, would support a diagnosis of acute or chronic glomerulonephritis or the nephrotic syndrome.

The glomerulus and the glomerular capsule

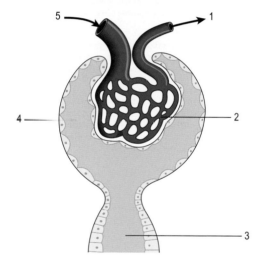

Fig 165

1. Efferent arteriole
2. Glomerulus
3. Proximal convoluted tubule
4. Glomerular capsule
5. Afferent arteriole

Comments

Anatomical: An afferent arteriole invaginates the glomerular capsule and divides into capillaries to form the glomerulus, from which the efferent arteriole exits.

Physiological: The renal arteries supply the kidneys with about 20% of the cardiac output. Filtration occurs across the semipermeable membranes of the glomerular capillaries and the glomerular capsule as a result of the pressure difference between the blood inside the glomerulus and the filtrate inside the glomerular capsule. Blood cells, plasma proteins and large molecules are not filtered. The glomerular filtrate has approximately the same composition as plasma. The volume of filtrate produced by the kidneys in 1 minute is the glomerular filtration rate (GFR). For adults, it is normally 125 mL/min, amounting to about 180 L/day. Only 1% will be excreted as urine because of tubular reabsorption.

Clinical: The average amount of urine passed daily varies between 1 and 1.5 litres. Its composition reflects renal function. Any change in renal function has an effect on the composition of urine, as, for example, its acid–base balance or electrolyte balance. The presence in the urine of blood cells, plasma proteins and large molecules, which are not normally filtered, is a sign of renal dysfunction. The colour and smell of urine depend on the concentration of the various substances and foods ingested. Renal insufficiency is defined as a significant reduction in the GFR and is graded according to the severity of the reduction. A GFR below 30 mL/min indicates severe renal insufficiency.

The ureters and their relations to the kidneys and the bladder

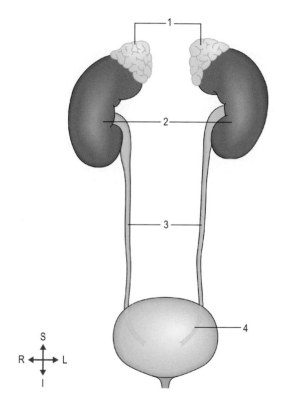

Fig 166

1. Suprarenal glands
2. Kidneys
3. Ureters
4. Bladder

Comments

Anatomical: The ureters, two in number, carry urine from the kidneys to the bladder. They measure about 25 cm in length and 3 mm in diameter. Their walls consist of three tissue layers — fibrous, muscular and mucosal. The funnel-shaped ureter is continuous with the renal pelvis. It descends in the abdominal and pelvic cavities and obliquely crosses the wall of the bladder, which is balloon-shaped and is an intrapelvic urine reservoir.

Physiological: The smooth muscle surrounding the ureter contracts to generate peristaltic waves to propel the urine towards the bladder in small spurts. The frequency of these contractions depends on the amount of urine to be moved.

Clinical: A urinary infection confined to the bladder is called *cystitis*. Its symptoms include a burning feeling on urination, a desire to pass urine frequently, difficulty in passing urine and bladder pain. In some cases, the infection reaches the kidney and becomes pyelonephritis, which can be complicated by a renal abscess and septicaemia.

The location of the ureter where it passes through the bladder wall

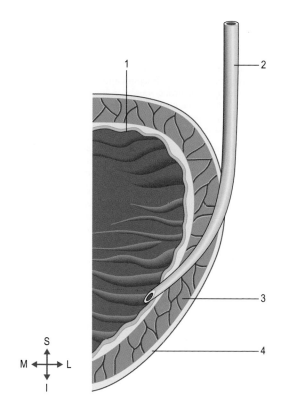

Fig 167

1. Bladder mucosa covered by transitional epithelium
2. Ureter
3. Layer of smooth muscle
4. Outer coat of the bladder wall (fibrous tissue)

Comments

Anatomical: The ureter consists of three tissue layers — an inner layer (a mucosa lined by transitional epithelium), a middle layer of smooth muscle and an outer layer made up of fibrous tissue and continuous with that of the kidney. It descends in the abdominal cavity and then in the pelvic cavity and runs obliquely through the wall of the bladder to open into its neck at the ureteric orifice.

Physiological: The urine is propelled in small spurts along the ureter by peristaltic activity of its smooth muscle. The spurt frequency depends on the volume of urine available. The internal ureteric sphincter, made up of smooth muscle, controls the passage of urine into the bladder; it is not under voluntary control. The oblique path through the bladder wall taken by the ureters ensures that their orifices into the bladder are closed when the bladder is full. This prevents reflux of urine from the bladder into the ureters and towards the kidneys when the bladder is filling or emptying.

Clinical: Vesicoureteric reflux can cause repeated renal infections and lead to chronic renal failure if left untreated.

Summary of the three stages of urine formation

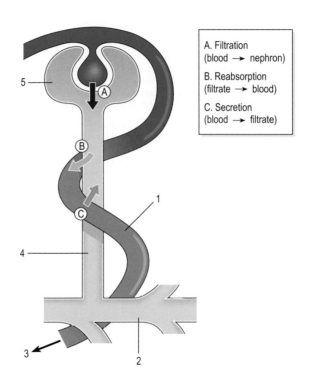

A. Filtration
(blood → nephron)

B. Reabsorption
(filtrate → blood)

C. Secretion
(blood → filtrate)

Fig 168

1. Capillary related to the nephron
2. Collecting duct
3. Towards the renal vein
4. Nephron
5. Glomerular capsule

Comments

Physiological: There are three processes involved in urine production — glomerular filtration, tubular reabsorption and tubular secretion. Filtration takes place during the passage of blood through the glomerulus. Tubular reabsorption of water and of electrolytes (e.g., sodium, potassium, calcium) is selective and occurs mainly in the proximal convoluted tubule. The balance between water intake and water loss is regulated by the kidneys. The amount of urine formed is controlled by the antidiuretic hormone, which is responsible for water reabsorption. Sodium excretion is controlled by the renin-angiotensin-aldosterone mechanism. When sodium reabsorption is enhanced, potassium excretion also increases. The kidneys play an important role in maintaining the body's water and electrolyte balance. Hydrogen ions are secreted by the tubules.

Clinical: At the end of urine formation, water is its main constituent. The normal composition of urine is 96% water, about 2% urea, less than 2% creatinine, ammonia, sodium and potassium and, finally, less than 2% chloride, phosphate, sulphate and oxalate. The urine volume has a mean value ranging from 1 to 1.5 L/day. The minimum volume of urine that must be excreted (the obligatory urine volume) is about 500 mL/day. Urine is clear and germ-free. It is amber-coloured as a result of the conversion of bilirubin to urobilin. Its pH is around 6. Oliguria, anuria, dysuria, nocturia, increase in urinary output (polyuria), increase in urinary frequency, haematuria, proteinuria, glycosuria and ketonuria are signs and symptoms of renal disease. The causes of renal insufficiency can be prerenal (e.g., disease of the renal arteries), renal or postrenal (e.g., for example, diseases of the ureter, bladder and prostate). When the cause is renal, it is classified according to the anatomical part responsible for the dysfunction (e.g., as disease of the glomeruli, the tubules, the interstitium and its blood vessels).

The pelvic organs adjacent to the bladder and the urethra in females

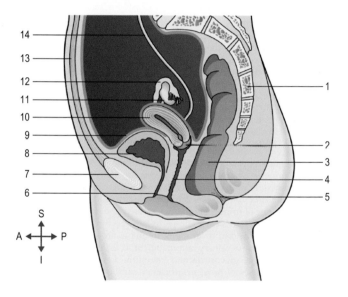

Fig 169

1. Sacrum
2. Uterine cervix
3. Rectum
4. Vagina
5. Anal canal
6. Urethra
7. Pubic bone
8. Bladder
9. Peritoneum
10. Uterus
11. Ovary
12. Fallopian tube
13. Anterior abdominal wall
14. Right ureter

Comments

Anatomical: The organs adjacent to the bladder in women are as follows: anteriorly, the pubic symphysis; posteriorly, the uterus and the upper part of the vagina; superiorly, the small intestine; inferiorly, the ureter and the muscles of the pelvic floor. The female urethra, which carries urine from the bladder to the exterior, measures about 4 cm in length and 6 mm in diameter.

Physiological: The urethral external orifice is controlled by the external urethral sphincter, which consists of striated muscle under voluntary control. A conscious effort allows it to contract to prevent urination.

Clinical: Cloudy, foul-smelling or blood-stained urine suggests an inflammatory disease of the urethra (urethritis), the bladder (cystitis) or the ureter (ureteritis). Women are more prone to these conditions because the female urethra is short and lies close to the perineum and the anus.

The pelvic organs adjacent to the bladder and the urethra in males

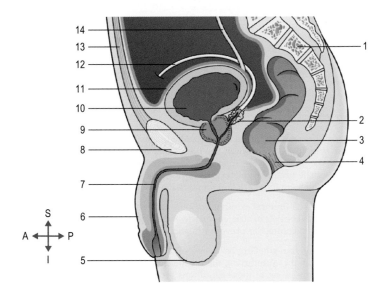

Fig 170

1. Sacrum
2. Seminal vesicle
3. Rectum
4. Anal canal
5. Scrotum
6. Penis
7. Urethra
8. Pubic bone
9. Prostate
10. Bladder
11. Peritoneum
12. Vas deferens
13. Anterior abdominal wall
14. Right ureter

Comments

Anatomical: The organs adjacent to the bladder in men are as follows: anteriorly, the pubic symphysis; posteriorly, the rectum and the seminal vesicles; superiorly, the small intestine; inferiorly, the urethra and the prostate. The male urethra, which carries urine from the bladder to the exterior, belongs to both the urinary and the reproductive systems. The male urethra is lined by a transitional epithelium, consisting of umbrella cells. Its length depends on that of the penis.

Physiological: The transitional epithelium is made up of umbrella cells that allow stretching to occur.

Clinical: Haematuria visible to the naked eye is known as *macroscopic haematuria*. In cases of what is called *microscopic haematuria*, the urine is clear, and the presence of blood is detected only on microscopic examination. Clinical signs and symptoms of disease or of infection of the urinary tract, such as urethritis, prostatitis or benign nodular prostatic hyperplasia include the following: dysuria (difficult urination in many stages, with stops and restarts, weak urine stream and uncontrolled leakage of a few drops of urine at the end of micturition); abnormally increased urinary frequency; urinary incontinence; a burning feeling on urination, especially at the level of the urethral meatus; purulent urethral discharge.

Section of the bladder showing the trigone

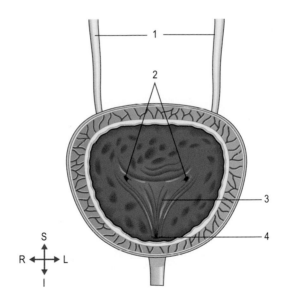

Fig 171

1. Ureters
2. Ureteric orifices
3. Trigone
4. Internal urethral orifice

Comments

Anatomical: When full, the bladder is like a balloon. It is partly covered by peritoneum. The three orifices in the bladder form a triangle, or trigone. The two upper orifices belong to the ureters and the third to the urethra. The bladder is continuous with the urethra at the bladder neck.

Physiological: The internal urethral sphincter controls the passage of urine from the bladder to the urethra; it is not under voluntary control.

Clinical: A normal urinary volume over 24 hours that is associated with a weak stream suggests urethral obstruction and prostatic enlargement. Urinary retention signifies total urethral obstruction caused by failure of the internal sphincter to open or by prostatic enlargement. Urine builds up in the bladder, which becomes distended into a globe, causing pain and an increase in the volume of the suprapubic region. The pain is due to the rapid stretching of the detrusor muscle. The distended bladder can occasionally contain 2 to 3 litres of urine and in older people it can manifest itself clinically only as a state of confusion.

Reflex control of micturition when a conscious effort fails to arrest the reflex to urinate

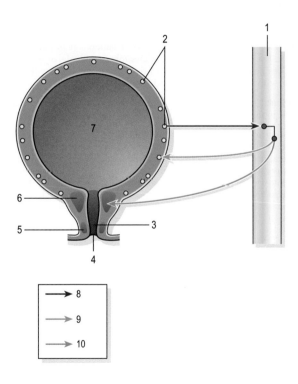

Fig 172

1. Spinal cord
2. Stretch-sensitive nerve endings
3. Urethra
4. External urethral orifice
5. External urethral sphincter
6. Internal urethral sphincter
7. Full bladder
8. Nerve impulses going to the spinal cord
9. Nerve impulses stimulating the contraction of the detrusor muscle
10. Nerve impulses causing the relaxation of the internal urethral sphincter

Comments

Anatomical: The bladder contains three openings, two related to the ureters and one to the urethra. It is continuous with the urethra at the bladder neck. Evacuation of urine from the bladder is regulated by the internal urethral sphincter and external urethral sphincter, with the latter being under voluntary control and the former not under voluntary control. The bladder is made up of three tissue layers. The outer layer consists of connective tissue, along with the blood vessels, lymphatics and nerves. The middle layer, which corresponds to the detrusor muscle, is made up of three layers of interlacing elastic and muscular fibres. The inner mucosal layer, lined by transitional epithelium and containing umbrella cells, forms a series of folds when the bladder is empty.

Physiological: Micturition is a reflex activity. As urine fills the bladder, the stretch receptors in the bladder are activated. The umbrella cells in the epithelium help the bladder to stretch. Sensory impulses are transmitted by afferent nerves to the spinal cord, and a spinal reflex results in the involuntary contraction of the detrusor muscle and involuntary relaxation of the internal urethral sphincter. Micturition takes place and the bladder is emptied of urine.

Clinical: The signs and symptoms of a distended bladder include pain in the hypogastrium, absence of urination for hours, a state of confusion and a state of agitation.

Control of micturition after bladder control is established

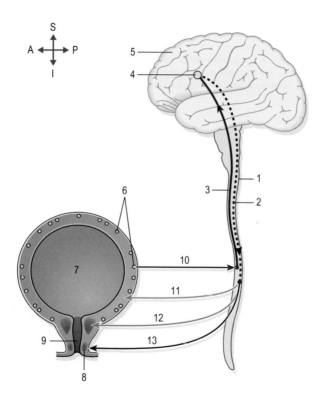

Fig 173

1. Spinal cord
2. Voluntary inhibition of the micturition reflex
3. Nerve impulse going to the cerebral cortex
4. Cerebral cortex
5. Brain
6. Stretch receptors
7. Full bladder
8. External urethral sphincter
9. Urethra
10. Nerve impulses going to the spinal cord
11. Nerve impulses stimulate contraction of the detrusor muscle
12. Nerve impulses stimulate relaxation of the internal urethral sphincter
13. A conscious effort to control the external urethral sphincter thwarts the micturition reflex

Comments

Anatomical: The internal urethral sphincter controls the evacuation of urine by an involuntary mechanism, whereas the external urethral sphincter exerts voluntary control over it. The middle layer of the bladder, the detrusor muscle, consists of three interlacing layers of elastic and muscle fibres.

Physiological: Micturition, which is the emptying of the bladder of urine, is a reflex action; however, it can be inhibited voluntarily by nervous signals sent to the cerebral cortex. Contraction of the external urethral sphincter and the muscles of the pelvic floor postpone micturition. This is the result of a learned voluntary act.

Clinical: The need to urinate is felt when the bladder volume is about 300 to 400 mL, whereas its capacity is about 600 mL. Control of micturition is the result of a learning process during the first few years of life. Incontinence is the involuntary passing of urine. Clinical observation and history taking can differentiate three types—stress incontinence, urge incontinence and overflow incontinence. Urinary incontinence, urinary urgency and increased urinary frequency raise the possibility of enuresis (bed wetting). Problems with micturition in the daytime are important in children. They can also be observed in those with neurological disorders, such as multiple sclerosis.

The skin

The main structures of the skin

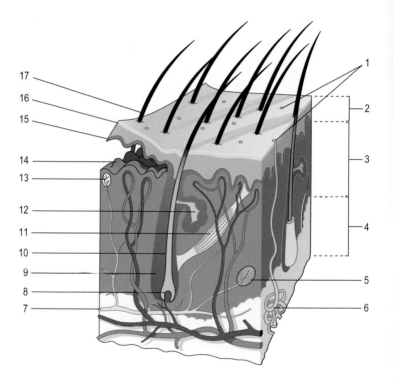

Fig 174

1. Openings of sweat ducts
2. Epidermis
3. Dermis
4. Subcutaneous tissue
5. Pacinian corpuscle
6. Sweat gland
7. Cutaneous nerve
8. Hair bulb
9. Hair follicle
10. Hair root
11. Arrector pili muscle
12. Sebaceous gland
13. Unencapsulated Meissner's corpuscle (tactile)
14. Dermal papilla
15. Basal layer
16. Cornified layer
17. Shaft of hair

Comments

Anatomical: The skin is the largest organ in the body, with a surface area of up to 2 m². It is made up of the epidermis, the dermis and the subcutaneous tissue. The epidermis is superficial and consists of a germinal basal layer and a thick keratinising layer. It contains no blood vessels or nerve endings. It is traversed by hairs, the secretory products of the sebaceous glands and the excretory ducts of the sweat glands. The papillae, which are upward projections of the dermis, come close to the surface. The dermis is made up of connective tissue containing collagen and elastic fibres responsible for its ability to be both strong and flexible. It contains blood vessels and lymphatics, nerve endings, sweat glands, sebaceous glands and hairs with their arrector pili muscles.

Physiological: The cells are produced in the basal layer and move up to the cornified layer. The basal layer has melanocytes, which secrete melanin when exposed to the sun. The dermal papillae allow the transfer of nutrients. The functions of the skin include protection of the body, control of body temperature, vitamin D synthesis, provision of sensory input and wound healing.

Clinical: A yellowish discolouration of the skin is due to the presence of blood-derived bile pigments or carotenoids in the subcutaneous fat. Stretch marks result from the stretching and subsequent rupture of the elastic fibres in cases of obesity or pregnancy. Skin lesions include macules, papules, vesicles, bullae, pustules, ulcers and nodules.

The sensory nerves of the dermis

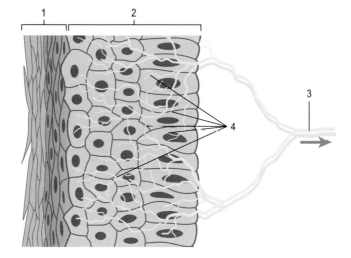

Fig 175

1. Epidermis
2. Dermis
3. Sensory nerve (transmitting sensory signals to the spinal cord and the brain)
4. Sensory nerve endings

Comments

Anatomical: The skin is a sensory organ. The dermis, lying between the epidermis and the subcutaneous tissue, contains specialised nerve endings sensitive to touch, temperature (cold or hot), pressure and pain.

Physiological: The nerve endings are the sensory receptors and are activated by different types of stimuli. If there are different types of stimuli, there are also various types of receptors sensitive to light pressure, strong pressure or pain. Nerve impulses are transmitted first by the sensory nerves to the spinal cord and then to the sensory areas of the brain.

Clinical: Any sensory loss is a clinical sign that deserves attention. In cases of damage to the dermis, as with a second-degree burn, the feeling of pain persists; however, this is lost in cases of third-degree burn because the sensory nerve endings have been destroyed.

The nail

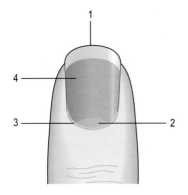

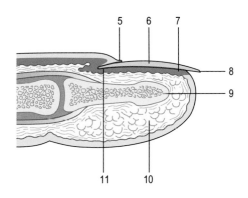

Fig 176

1. Free nail edge
2. Lunule
3. Cuticle
4. Nail plate
5. Cuticle
6. Nail
7. Nail bed
8. Free nail edge
9. Distal phalanx
10. Subcutaneous fat
11. Nail root

Comments

Anatomical: The nails, the epidermis and the hairs are derived from the same type of cells.

Physiological: The nail grows from the basal layer of the epidermis, which is the nail bed. The cuticle, covering the nail, becomes the lunule, which is a white patch continuous with the nail plate and the free nail end. Consisting of a plate of cornified keratin, the nail protects the extremities of the fingers and the toes.

Clinical: Fingernails grow faster than toenails, and their growth rate increases as the temperature rises. Signs of disease of the nails include changes in nail colour, such as whitening or yellowing at their lateral margins or at their distal edges, as well as any sign of brittleness, looseness or thickening. Clubbing of the fingers, due to a deformation of the nails, which become rounded and shiny like a watch glass, is mostly observed during the progression of some lung diseases, such as tumours and fibrotic disorders of the lung, but also with some gastrointestinal diseases (e.g., Crohn's disease, ulcerative colitis, cirrhosis of the liver) and some cardiac conditions.

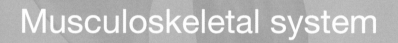

Musculoskeletal system

A long bone, partially sectioned

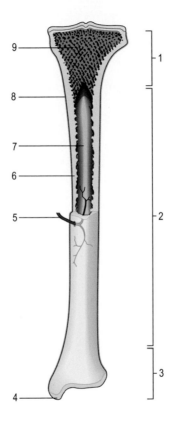

Fig 177

1. Epiphysis
2. Diaphysis (shaft)
3. Epiphysis
4. Articular (hyaline) cartilage
5. Nutrient artery entering its nutrient foramen
6. Compact bone
7. Medullary cavity (contains yellow marrow)
8. Periosteum
9. Spongy bone (contains red marrow)

Comments

Anatomical: A long bone consists of a shaft or diaphysis and two extremities, or epiphyses, and is covered by a vascular membrane, or periosteum. The shaft is made up of compact bone, with a medullary cavity filled with bone marrow. The epiphyses consist of spongy bone coated with compact bone. The shaft is separated from the epiphyses by the epiphyseal cartilages. In the joint, the periosteum is replaced by hyaline cartilage. The shaft is supplied by nutrient arteries and the epiphyses by a capillary network. The sensory nerves enter the bone near the nutrient artery and then divide to spread into the entire bone.

Physiological: One of the two layers of the periosteum has a protective role; the other contains osteoblasts and osteoclasts, which take part in remodelling the bone. The osteoblasts form bone; the osteoclasts break it down.

Clinical: In cases of trauma or a bony lesion, pain is a warning sign that allows the lesion to be localised and diagnosed. The pain is acute and can become chronic as a result of secondary factors, such as anxiety, sleep disturbances, difficulty moving the affected bone, posttraumatic lesions and damage to nerves.

Sections of a flat bone and an irregular bone

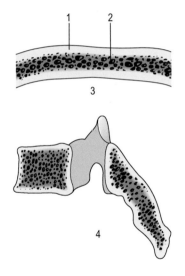

Fig 178

374

1. Compact bone
2. Spongy bone
3. Flat bone (e.g., cranial bone)
4. Irregular bone (e.g., vertebra)

Comments

Anatomical: Flat and irregular bones have different shapes; neither of them has a shaft or an epiphysis. The bone is made up of hard and resistant connective tissue packed essentially with calcium salts. The osteoclasts are located under the periosteum and around the medullary cavity.

Physiological: The bone cells—the osteoblasts and the osteoclasts—have different functions. The osteoblasts form bone by depositing bone salts in the bony tissue. Osteoclasts break down and release calcium and phosphate. The balance between these two activities keeps the bone healthy. Osteocytes are involved in its maintenance.

Clinical: When a bone is fractured, the osteoclasts promote healing and repair by maintaining and canalising the callus.

Microstructure of compact bone

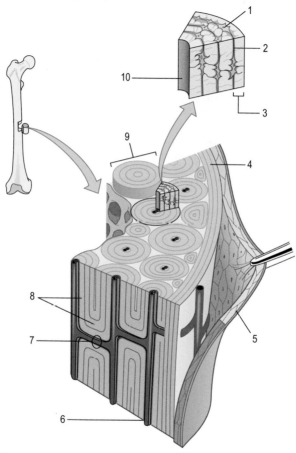

Fig 179

1. Lacuna with osteocytes
2. Canaliculus
3. Lamellae
4. Circumferential lamellae
5. Periosteum (detached)
6. Central canal (haversian)
7. Volkmann's canal
8. Lamellae
9. Osteon (haversian system)
10. Central canal (haversian)

Comments

Anatomical: Compact bone is made up of parallel tubular structures, called *osteons* or *haversian systems*, which are responsible for its great resistance. Their central canals contain blood vessels, lymphatics and nerves, and they are linked to one another by Volkmann's canals. The lamellae are cylindrical sheets of bone arranged around the central canals and, among them, there are cavities, with each containing an osteocyte.

Physiological: An osteocyte is a mature bone cell that controls and preserves the bone. It is fed by the interstitial fluid in the canaliculi, which comes from the central canal of the osteon.

Clinical: The total bone mass of the body consists of 80% compact bone. In the femur, the osteons run from one epiphysis to the other.

Microstructure of spongy bone

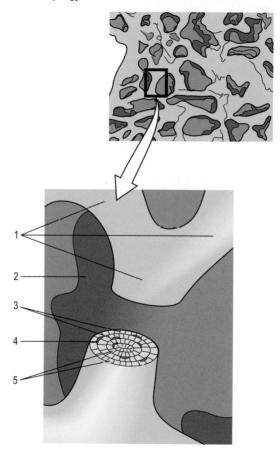

Fig 180

1. Lamellae
2. Space for the red marrow
3. Canaliculi
4. Osteocytes
5. Trabeculae

Comments

Anatomical: Spongy bone is made up of trabeculae, which are sheets of bone, and osteocytes, linked by canaliculi. The spaces between these trabeculae contain red marrow.

Physiological: The osteocytes are nourished by the interstitial fluid, which permeates the bone via the canaliculi.

Clinical: Because it is lighter than compact bone, spongy bone decreases the weight of the bony skeleton.

Developmental stages of a long bone

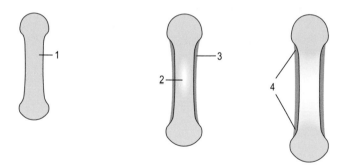

Fig 181 Fetal development

1. Cartilaginous precursor
2. Site of primary ossification
3. Periosteal collar
4. Elongation of the diaphysis

Comments

Physiological: During fetal development, ossification of the long bones begins in areas containing osteogenic cells, and called *centres of ossification*. With progressive vascularisation, the cartilage will be transformed into bone. The osteoblasts secrete the components of bone into the diaphysis. By the 8th week of gestation, a periosteal collar develops. The bone grows in length, and the process of ossification keeps up with its growth and extends to both epiphyses.

Clinical: In osteogenesis imperfecta, the developmental process of ossification is abnormal, leading to the formation of fragile bones and a higher rate of bone fractures. For this reason, osteogenesis imperfecta is known as the *brittle bone disease*.

Developmental stages of a long bone

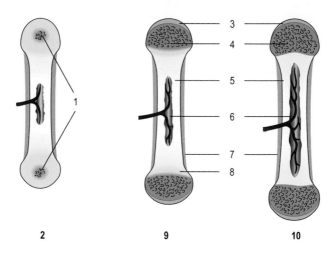

Fig 182

1. Centres of secondary ossification in the epiphyses
2. At birth
3. Hyaline cartilage
4. Spongy bone
5. Compact bone
6. Medullary cavity
7. Periosteum
8. Epiphyseal cartilage
9. Childhood and adolescence
10. Adulthood

Comments

Physiological: Ossification of bone proceeds as the bone increases in length. The bony tissue is built and remodelled constantly. During childhood, the epiphyseal plate at each extremity of the bone produces cartilage where it is in contact with the diaphysis. Pituitary and thyroid hormones stimulate the growth of a long bone and control its size and shape. Calcitonin and parathormone regulate the deposition and resorption of calcium in bones, respectively. Bones get thicker without growing indefinitely. At puberty, the increase in sex hormone levels (testosterone and oestrogen) promotes bone growth and also stops it by stimulating the closure of the epiphyseal plates. Under the influence of these hormones, the epiphyseal plate stops growing, and the bone stops increasing in length.

Clinical: Men are taller than women because male puberty has a later onset. Osteoporosis is the weakening of bones; it usually occurs after menopause in women because of the drop in blood levels of oestrogens, which play an important role in maintaining bone mass in the body. It predisposes to the risk of fractures, notably of the femoral neck, the vertebrae and the lower extremity of the radius.

Stages of bone repair

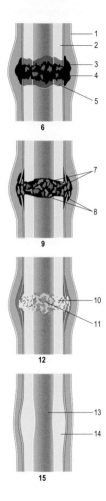

Fig 183

1. Periosteum
2. Compact bone
3. Haematoma
4. Fragments of dead bone
5. Local inflammatory response
6. Formation of a haematoma
7. Deposition of cartilage and of spongy bone by osteoblasts (callus)
8. Fragments of dead bone and tissue removed by phagocytes
9. Start of callus formation
10. Continuous formation of callus and patches of spongy bone—unites the extremities of the fracture
11. Progressive removal of the haematoma
12. Ends of the bone are reunited
13. Recanalisation of the medullary cavity by osteoclasts
14. Replacement of the spongy bone by compact bone
15. Recanalisation and normalisation of the structure of the bone

Comments

Physiological: There are four phases in the healing of a fracture. The first is the formation of the haematoma between the two ends of the bone and the surrounding soft tissues. The second is the formation of the callus. An acute inflammatory process produces an exudate containing macrophages, which phagocytose the haematoma and the fragments of dead bone. The fibroblasts then move in and form granulation tissue and new capillaries. The osteoblasts secrete spongy bone. New deposits of bone and cartilage give rise to the callus. The third phase occurs when the two ends of the fractured bone are reunited. At the end of many weeks, the callus matures, and bone replaces cartilage. In the fourth phase, the bone is re-formed, and the medullary cavity is recanalised across the callus.

Clinical: A stress or fatigue fracture can occur during a bout of unusual physical activity or during overtraining. Fractures are called *simple* if their broken ends do not pierce the skin, *open* if the bones jut out and *pathological* if the bone involved is defective because of some disease process. Misalignment of the two ends of the bone during the remodelling phase can lead to a permanent disability. A bone infection is called *osteomyelitis*. A hard, bony outgrowth, whether asymptomatic or painful on mechanical irritation, can be a sign of one of the exostosis syndromes.

The skeleton (1), anterior view

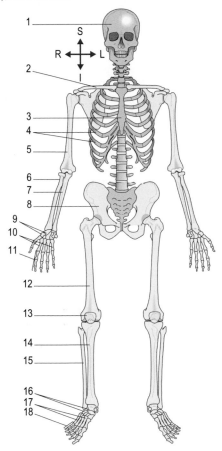

Fig 184 The axial skeleton is in *yellow*; the appendicular skeleton is in *light brown*.

1. Cranium
2. Clavicle
3. Sternum
4. Ribs
5. Humerus
6. Radius
7. Ulna
8. Pelvis
9. Carpal bones
10. Metacarpal bones
11. Phalanges
12. Femur
13. Patella
14. Tibia
15. Fibula
16. Tarsal bones
17. Metatarsal bones
18. Phalanges

Comments

Anatomical: The body skeleton, composed of 206 bones, is divided into many parts. The axial skeleton forms the central axis of the body and is made up of the cranium, the vertebral column, the ribs and the sternum. The appendicular skeleton consists of the shoulders, the pelvic girdle and the limb bones.

Physiological: Depending on their anatomical location, bones take part in movements and the protection of organs.

Clinical: The fetal skeleton is cartilaginous, ossification starts before birth and continues until adulthood. The dry mass of the skeleton without red marrow is higher in men, 5 kg; it is 3 kg in women. Some people may have one bone too many. In cases of physical trauma, a clinical examination includes looking for pain and for partial or total loss of function, the site of the lesion and evidence of failure of the respiratory, vascular or nervous system.

The skeleton (2), lateral view

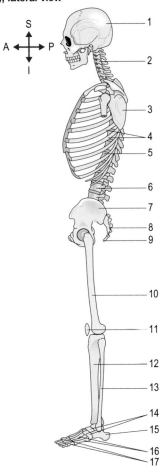

Fig 185

1. Cranium
2. Cervical vertebrae
3. Scapula
4. Ribs
5. Thoracic vertebrae
6. Lumbar vertebra
7. Pelvis
8. Sacrum
9. Coccyx
10. Femur
11. Patella
12. Tibia
13. Fibula
14. Tarsal bones
15. Calcaneus
16. Metatarsal bones
17. Phalanges

Comments

Anatomical: The axial skeleton is made up of the head, the vertebral column, the ribs and the sternum. The vertebral column has 26 bones; 24 of them are separate vertebrae located between the occipital bone and the sacrum. It is subdivided into segments; the cervical segment has seven vertebrae, the thoracic segment has twelve vertebrae and the lumbar segment has five vertebrae. The sacrum results from the fusion of five vertebrae; the coccyx results from the fusion of three or four vertebrae. The appendicular skeleton is comprised of the shoulders, the pelvic girdle and the limb bones.

Physiological: The functions of the skeleton are to provide a frame for the body, allow movements to take place and protect some organs, such as the heart and lungs in the thoracic cage and the brain inside the cranium. Most of the organs lie inside the skeleton.

Clinical: Depending on its location, a bone fracture can cause respiratory, vascular or neurological problems. The clinical picture would suggest looking specifically for an open wound, for a haematoma undergoing more or less progressive resorption, for oedema, with the risk of nerve compression, and for multiple contusions.

The cranial bones and their sutures (joints)

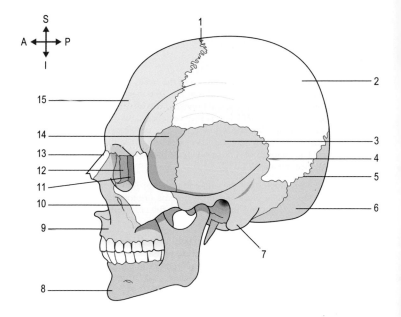

Fig 186

1. Coronal suture
2. Parietal bone
3. Temporal bone
4. Squamosal suture
5. Lambdoid suture
6. Occipital bone
7. Mastoid process
8. Mandible
9. Maxillary
10. Zygomatic bone
11. Lacrimal bone
12. Ethmoid bone
13. Nasal bone
14. Sphenoid bone
15. Frontal bone

Comments

Anatomical: The cranium consists of eight flat or irregular bones that protect the brain—the frontal bone, the occipital bone, the sphenoid bone, the ethmoid bone, the two parietal and the two temporal bones. Their periosteum is formed by a layer of the dura mater. The coronal suture unites the frontal and the two parietal bones, the sagittal suture unites the parietal bones, the lambdoid suture unites the parietal and occipital bones, and the squamosal suture unites the parietal and temporal bones. The nerves, the blood vessels and the lymphatics go through perforations, or foramina. In adults, the articulations between these bones are fixed. The zygomatic bone is the cheekbone, the maxillary bone is that of the upper jaw and the mandible is that of the lower jaw.

Clinical: Transient loss of consciousness and attention disturbances can be seen in cases of concussion due to a blow to the head. In cases of cerebral contusion with haemorrhage or oedema, there are neurological disturbances that correspond to the site of the lesion.

The bones of the cranial base and the cranial fossae, seen from above

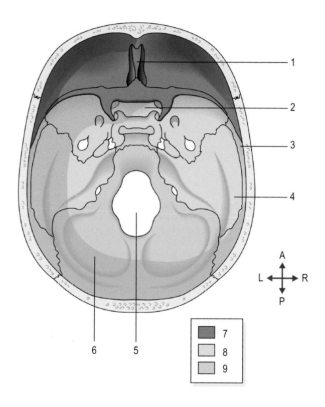

Fig 187

1. Ethmoid bone
2. Sphenoid bone
3. Right parietal bone
4. Right temporal bone
5. Foramen magnum
6. Occipital bone
7. Anterior cranial fossa
8. Middle cranial fossa
9. Posterior cranial fossa

Comments

Anatomical: There are three cranial fossae. The anterior fossa is made up of the ethmoid and frontal bones, the middle fossa is made up of the sphenoid, parietal and temporal bones, and the posterior fossa is made up of the occipital bone. The ethmoid bone forms part of the orbital cavity, the nasal cavity and the nasal septum. The frontal bone forms part of the orbital cavities. The foramen magnum allows the spinal cord to pass through. The olfactory nerve runs along the ethmoid bone, and the optic nerve goes through the optic foramen of the sphenoid.

Physiological: The orbits protect the eyes and provide sites of attachment for the muscles that move them.

Clinical: The leakage of clear fluid from the nose and the loss of cerebrospinal fluid through the ears suggest a fracture at the base of the cranium associated with the presence of fistulae between the meninges, nasal cavities, and middle ear, respectively. In cases of head trauma, neurological signs and symptoms may include pain, loss of consciousness, coma, disorientation in time and space, mental clouding, agitation or drowsiness, loss of feeling and motor paralysis. Loss of consciousness can cause respiratory problems or the aspiration of gastric contents, culminating in a medical emergency. Headaches, nosebleeds, partial loss of visual acuity, progressive loss of eye movements, facial neuralgia or paralysis, partial hearing loss, vertigo and problems with balance or swallowing are potential indications of tumours at the cranial base.

The right temporal bone, lateral view

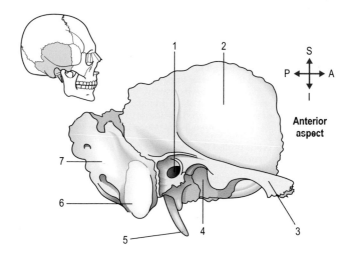

S

P ← → A

I

Anterior
aspect

Fig 188

1. External acoustic meatus
2. Squamous part
3. Zygomatic process
4. Site of the temporomandibular joint
5. Styloid process
6. Mastoid process
7. Mastoid part

Comments

Anatomical: The zygomatic process and the zygomatic bone make up the zygomatic arch. The styloid process provides attachment sites for the muscles of the tongue and the pharynx. The mastoid process, lying behind the ear, contains cavities that communicate with it. The petrous part of the temporal bone contains the organs of hearing and balance. The acoustic meatus is located close to the temporomandibular joint. The squamous part of the bone is thin and fan-shaped.

Physiological: The temporal bone, which protects the structures of the inner ear, and the mandible unite to form the temporomandibular joint (TMJ), where movements of the mandible can take place. The mandible is responsible for swallowing, chewing, phonation and yawning.

Clinical: Muscle pains, a cracking sound heard on opening or closing the TMJ, tinnitus, supersensitive hearing, earache, vertigo and sensation of blocked ears suggest TMJ disease. Loss of hearing, pain and the rapid onset of a high fever with shivering raise the possibility of mastoiditis. Signs of a rise in intracranial pressure (e.g., disturbance of consciousness), a clinical picture suggestive of a lesion of the temporal lobe (e.g., coma, paralysis), signs of a focal cerebral lesion (e.g., hemiparesis, focal seizures) and a lesion of the brainstem (e.g., ventilatory or haemodynamic disturbances) suggest the presence of a subdural haematoma.

The occipital bone, seen from below

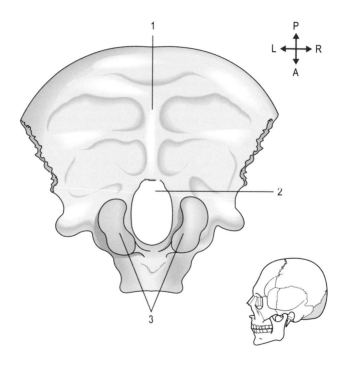

Fig 189

1. External occipital protuberance
2. Foramen magnum
3. Condyles for articulation with the atlas

Comments

Anatomical: The occipital bone forms the back of the head and part of the cranial base. Its concave internal surface harbours the occipital lobes and the cerebellum.

Physiological: The occipital bone and the atlas together form the bicondylar joint, which allows bending movements of the head to occur. The foramen magnum allows the spinal cord to enter the cranium.

Clinical: The term *joint* refers to all forms of union between two parts of the skeleton without necessarily implying any notion of mobility. The joints that unite the cranial bones are fixed.

The sphenoid bone, seen from above

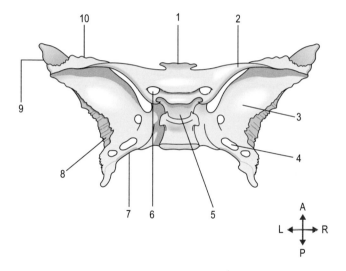

Fig 190

1. Articular facet for the ethmoid
2. Lesser wing
3. Greater wing
4. Foramen ovale
5. Pituitary fossa
6. Optic foramen
7. Articular facet for the occipital bone
8. Articular facet for the temporal bone
9. Articular facet for the parietal bone
10. Articular facet for the frontal bone

Comments

Anatomical: The butterfly-shaped sphenoid bone occupies the middle part of the cranial base. It articulates with the occipital, temporal, parietal, frontal and ethmoid bones. It links the cranial bones to the facial bones. The hypophyseal fossa, or sella turcica, contains the pituitary gland.

Physiological: The optic foramen allows the passage of the optic nerve, and the foramen ovale allows the passage of the mandibular nerve (a branch of the trigeminal nerve).

Clinical: Severe headaches behind the eye and a high fever suggest sphenoid sinusitis. If the symptoms persist beyond 2 weeks, the sinusitis is termed *chronic*; otherwise it is termed *acute*.

The right nasal cavity, left lateral view

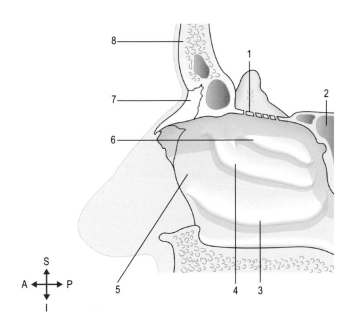

Fig 191

1. Cribriform plate of the ethmoid bone
2. Sphenoidal sinus
3. Inferior nasal concha
4. Middle nasal concha (ethmoidal)
5. Maxillary bone
6. Superior nasal concha (ethmoidal)
7. Nasal bone
8. Frontal bone

Comments

Anatomical: The frontal bone forms part of the orbital cavities and the supraorbital margin. One of its sinuses opens into the nasal cavity. The ethmoid bone contributes to the formation of the orbital cavity, the nasal septum, the lateral walls of the nasal cavity and the superior and middle nasal conchae. It also contains air sinuses that open into the nasal cavity via the cribriform plate in its roof. The nasal bones are two flat bones making up the bulk of the nasal bridge. The horizontally curved inferior conchae form the walls of the nasal cavity.

Physiological: By increasing the surface area of the nasal cavity, the conchae warm up and humidify the respired air.

Clinical: Facial pain, diffuse headache, fever, nasal congestion and sneezing are the typical symptoms of sinusitis. The nasal secretions can be purulent (greenish-yellow in colour) or transparent in cases of viral sinusitis. An acute sinusitis lasts about 2 weeks. The signs and symptoms of frontal sinusitis and ethmoidal sinusitis are different; a pounding pain above the eye, high fever and a runny nose on one side suggest the former, whereas swelling of one eyelid, pain at the level of the eye and a temperature above 38.5°C suggest the latter.

The facial bones, anterior view

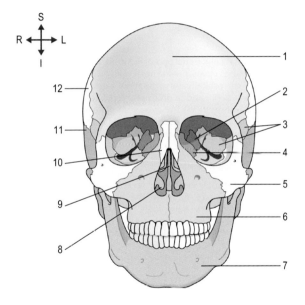

Fig 192

1. Frontal bone
2. Ethmoid bone
3. Sphenoid bone
4. Lacrimal bone
5. Zygomatic bone
6. Maxilla
7. Mandible
8. Inferior nasal concha
9. Vomer
10. Nasal bone
11. Temporal bone
12. Parietal bone

Comments

Anatomical: The facial skeleton is comprised of 14 bones: the frontal bone, two zygomatic bones (cheekbones), two nasal bones (confined to the nose), two palatine bones, two lacrimal bones, two inferior nasal conchae, the maxilla (the bone of the upper jaw), the vomer and the mandible (the bone of the lower jaw). The L-shaped palatine bones form part of the palate and the lateral wall of the nasal cavity. The flat nasal bones form the lateral and superior borders of the nasal bridge.

Physiological: The mandible (the bone of the lower jaw) is the only mobile bone in the head. The mandible and the maxilla contain the alveolar processes, where the teeth are implanted. The mandible, the site of attachment of muscles and ligaments, forms part of the temporomandibular joint. The ethmoid bone protects the eyes and gives attachment to the muscles that move them.

Clinical: The diagnostic features of a broken nose include pain, mobility and swelling of the nose, with or without distortion of the nasal septum. A runny nose, a stuffy nose or an itchy nose suggests a rhinitis.

The left mandible, lateral view

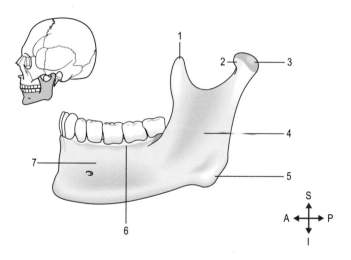

Fig 193

404

1. Coronoid process
2. Condylar process
3. Articular facet for the temporomandibular joint
4. Ramus
5. Angle
6. Alveolar process
7. Body

Comments

Anatomical: The bone of the mandible (the lower jaw) is made up of two parts joined by a median line to form a curved body that contains the teeth embedded in its alveolar process and a ramus, which divides to form the condylar process and the coronoid process. The former contacts the temporal bone to form the temporomandibular joint (TMJ); the latter is a site of attachment for muscles and ligaments. The angle of the mandible lies between its body and its ramus.

Physiological: The mandible is the only mobile bone in the head. The alveolar process lodges the teeth, and the coronoid process is the site of attachment of muscles and ligaments and forms part of the TMJ.

Clinical: The signs and symptoms of a mandibular fracture include pain when moving the mandible, pain during mastication, bleeding from the mouth, drooling (sialorrhea), and trismus (constant involuntary contractions of the jaw muscles).

The cranium with its fontanelles and sutures

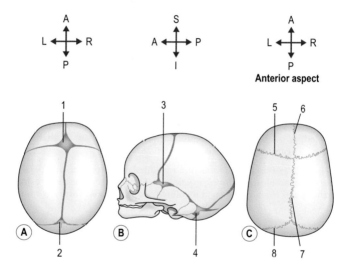

Fig 194 (A) Fontanelles, seen from above. **(B)** Fontanelles, seen from the side.
(C) Main sutures fully ossified, seen from above.

1. Anterior fontanelle
2. Posterior fontanelle
3. Sphenoidal fontanelle
4. Mastoid fontanelle
5. Coronal suture
6. Frontal suture
7. Sagittal suture
8. Lambdoid suture

Comments

Anatomical: At birth the cranial sutures are present but not yet ossified, to allow moulding of the baby's head during labour. The fontanelles are membranes that link together many of the cranial bones.

Physiological: The posterior and anterior fontanelles ossify by 3 months and by 12 to 18 months of age, respectively.

Clinical: Depression of the fontanelles is a sign of dehydration. Conversely, a bulging fontanelle suggests an intracranial space-occupying process associated with a subdural haematoma, meningitis or encephalitis. Failure of the fontanelles to close after 18 months is a sign of congenital hypothyroidism (cretinism) or of rickets.

The vertebral column, lateral view

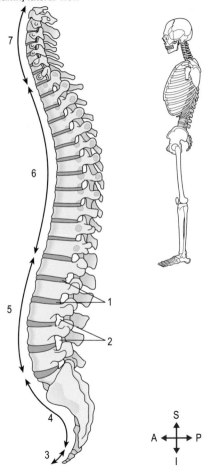

Fig 195

1. Intervertebral discs
2. Intervertebral foramina
3. Coccyx
4. Sacrum
5. Lumbar vertebrae (5)
0. Thoracic vertebrae (12)
7. Cervical vertebrae (7)

Comments

Anatomical: The vertebral column is made up of 26 bones — 24 vertebrae, the sacrum and the coccyx. The seven cervical vertebrae make up the cervical region, the 12 thoracic vertebrae make up the thoracic region, and the five lumbar vertebrae make up the lumbar region. Five vertebrae fuse to form the sacrum and four fuse to form the coccyx. The intervertebral disc is a cushion-like fibrocartilaginous structure that prevents direct contact between the bones. The vertebral foramina form the spinal canal, in which the spinal cord is lodged.

Physiological: The vertebral column acts as a bony protector of the fragile spinal cord. The vertebral foramina cooperate to form the spinal canal and the intervertebral discs act as shock absorbers. The column supports the head, maintains the axis of the trunk and allows movements to occur.

Clinical: Each vertebra is identified by the first letter of the region of the column to which it belongs, followed by a number, which indicates its location. Kyphosis and lordosis are deformities of the vertebral column characterised, respectively, by an excessive posterior convexity and an excessive anterior convexity.

A lumbar vertebra showing the features of a typical vertebra, seen from above

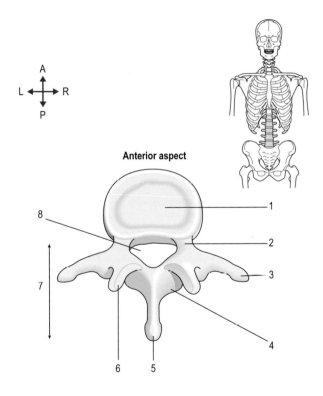

A
L ← → R
P

Anterior aspect

8

1

2

3

7

4

6   5

Fig 196

410

1. Body
2. Pedicle
3. Transverse process
4. Lamina
5. Spinous process
6. Superior articular process
7. Vertebral arch
8. Vertebral foramen

Comments

Anatomical: A vertebra is made up of a vertebral body attached to a vertebral arch by two pedicles. The body constitutes the bulk of the vertebra. The vertebrae articulate with each other at the level of their flat bodies, which nevertheless are not in contact because of the intervening intervertebral discs. The vertebral arch encloses the vertebral foramen; its walls consist of pedicles and bony laminae and allow the passage of the spinal cord. There are three processes — the transverse, the spinous and the articular.

Physiological: The bodies of the lumbar vertebrae are bulkier in size than the others to be able to support the body's weight. The spinous processes stick out to give attachment to muscles. Flexion (bending forward), extension (bending backward), lateral flexion (bending to one side) and rotation are movements that occur mostly in the cervical and lumbar regions.

Clinical: Lumbago, or pain in the lumbar region, suggests the presence of arthritis or degenerative changes in the discs. Pain, sphincter disturbances and neurological signs and symptoms, including paraplegia, are suggestive of spinal cord compression, characterised by motor and sensory deficits related to the level of compression.

A cervical vertebra showing its typical features, seen from above

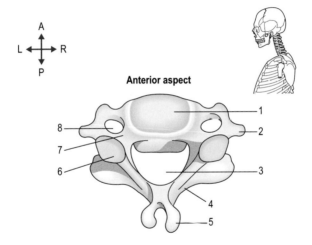

Anterior aspect

Fig 197

412

1. Body
2. Transverse process
3. Vertebral foramen
4. Lamina
5. Bifid spinous process
6. Articular process with a facet (in *blue*) for the adjacent vertebra
7. Pedicle
8. Foramen transversarium for the vertebral artery

Comments

Anatomical: The cervical vertebrae are the smallest bones in the column. The first two, the atlas and the axis, are different from the other five (C3–C7), which share similar features. Their bodies are small, their vertebral foramina are larger than those of the others, and their spinous processes are bifid, with two extremities. Their transverse processes contain foramina transversaria, which allow the vertebral artery (a branch of the subclavian artery) to travel up to the brain.

Physiological: Their movements include flexion (bending forward), extension (bending backward), lateral flexion (bending to one side) and rotation.

Clinical: The seventh cervical vertebra (C7) has a prominent spinous process in the shape of a bulbous tubercle, which can be felt at the base of the neck. The risk of dislocation is highest in the cervical region because the articular facets of these vertebrae are more horizontal and do not fit together as well. The width of the vertebral canal in this region allows a minor dislocation to occur without any damage to the cord, which can, however, take place in cases of severe dislocation or fracture.

The atlas, the first cervical vertebra, seen from above

Anterior aspect

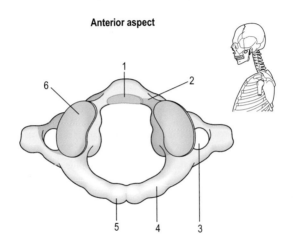

Fig 198

414

1. Articular facet for the dens (odontoid process) of the axis
2. Pedicle
3. Foramen transversarium for the vertebral artery
4. Lamina
5. Posterior tubercle equivalent to the spinous process
6. Articular facet for the occipital condyle

Comments

Anatomical: The first cervical vertebra, the atlas or C1, according to nomenclature used for naming the vertebrae, is a bony ring on which the head rests. It lies above the axis (C2) and is made up of an anterior arch and a posterior arch fused together. It bears two flat facets on its superior aspect and two short transverse processes perforated by the foramen transversarium, which is a passage for the vertebral artery on its way to the brain. It has neither a body nor a spinous process.

Physiological: The facets form condylar joints with the occipital bone and the axis, allowing movements of head flexion and extension to occur.

Clinical: As the effects of a traumatic injury to the atlas are regressing, a search for vascular signs and symptoms will help establish the diagnosis of the lesions involved

The axis, the second cervical vertebra, seen from above

Anterior aspect

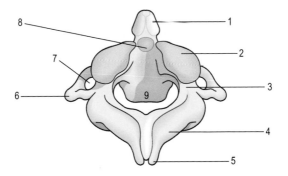

Fig 199

1. Dens (odontoid process)
2. Facet for the atlas
3. Pedicle
4. Lamina
5. Spinous process
6. Transverse process
7. Foramen transversarium for the vertebral artery
8. Facet for the transverse ligament
9. Body

Comments

Anatomical: The axis, or C2, according to the nomenclature used for vertebrae, is the second cranial vertebra, which lies below the atlas. It has a small body with a structure projecting upwards, which is called the *dens* or *odontoid process* and that partly fills the posterior foramen of the atlas and makes contact with the transverse ligament.

Physiological: By articulating with the atlas, the axis allows the head to be rotated from side to side.

Clinical. As the effects of a traumatic injury to the axis are receding, looking for vascular signs and symptoms will help establish the diagnosis of the lesions involved.

The atlas and the axis in place together with the transverse ligament, seen from above

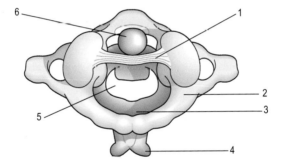

Fig 200

1. Transverse ligament
2. Atlas
3. Axis
4. Spinous process of axis
5. Vertebral foramen
6. Dens (odontoid process) of axis

Comments

Anatomical: The atlas (C1) and the axis (C2) are the first two cervical vertebrae. The axis has a structure projecting upwards, the dens, which articulates anteriorly with the bony part of the atlas and posteriorly with the ligamentous portion of the ring of the atlas. These two vertebrae are linked by the transverse ligament, which articulates with the posterior surface of the dens of the axis.

Physiological: There are three synovial atlantoaxial joints. The two lateral joints are between the lateral masses of the two vertebrae. The median joint is a pivot joint between the dens of the axis and the anterior arch of the atlas. These joints allow the head to be rotated from side to side.

A thoracic vertebra

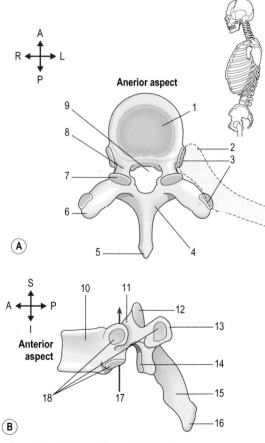

Anerior aspect

Anterior aspect

Fig 201 **(A)** Seen from above. **(B)** Seen from the side.

(A) Seen from above

1. Body
2. Head of rib
3. Articular facets for ribs
4. Lamina
5. Spinous process
6. Transverse process
7. Articular process with articular facet for adjacent rib
8. Pedicle
9. Vertebral foramen

(B) Seen from the side

10. Body
11. Pedicle
12. Superior articular process with articular facet for adjacent rib
13. Transverse process
14. Inferior articular process
15. Lamina
16. Spinous process
17. Arrow going through the vertebral foramen
18. Articular facets for the ribs

Comments

Anatomical: The 12 thoracic vertebrae have the same features as the cervical vertebrae, but are larger in size to be able to support more weight. The body and the processes have articular facets for the ribs (costal facets). There are three processes that protrude — the transverse, the spinous and the articular processes. The vertebral foramen is a hole between the vertebral pedicles, protecting and allowing the passage of spinal nerves, blood vessels and lymphatics.

Physiological: There are limited movements between the vertebrae of the vertebral column, including flexion (bending forward), extension (bending backward), lateral flexion (bending to one side) and rotation.

Clinical: Lateral deviation of the vertebral column suggests a diagnosis of scoliosis. The signs and symptoms of a vertebral tumour include variably severe localised pain that is made worse by lying down and is absent during walking and also as a result of neurological deficits.

The sacrum and the coccyx

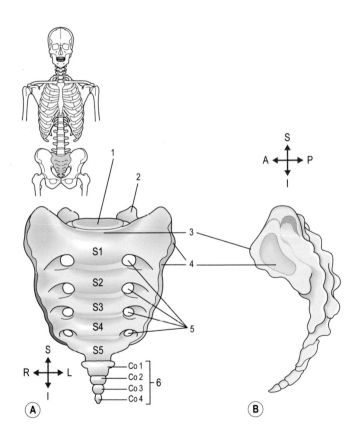

Fig 202 (A) Anterior aspect. **(B)** Lateral aspect.

1. Articular surface for the intervertebral disc
2. Articular process for L5
3. Promontory
4. Articular facets for the left iliac bone
5. Foramina for the passage of nerves
6. Coccyx

Comments

Anatomical: The sacrum and the coccyx, both triangular in shape, consist respectively of five and four fused vertebrae. The sacrum articulates with the 5th lumbar vertebra (L5), the iliac bones and the coccyx. The sacral promontory is one of the projections into the pelvic cavity and gives rise to the sacroiliac joints on both sides. The vertebral foramina are present as in all other vertebrae, and the spinal nerves exit through them in sequential fashion. The coccyx articulates with the distal apex of the sacrum.

Clinical: The sacroiliac joints can be involved by an arthritic process as part of one of the spondyloarthropathies. The patient has low back pain that is consistent with an inflammatory process and is associated with waking up at night and with morning stiffness that is relieved by movement. In advanced stages, an x-ray shows fusion of the edges of the sacroiliac joints.

Section of the vertebral column showing the ligaments, the intervertebral discs and the intervertebral foramina, anterior view

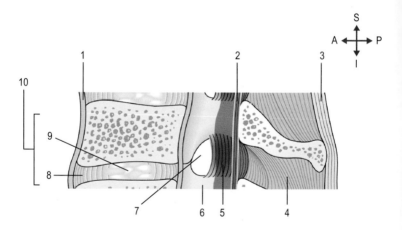

Fig 203

1. Anterior longitudinal ligament
2. Posterior longitudinal ligament
3. Supraspinous ligament
4. Interspinous ligament
5. Ligamentum flavum
6. Vertebral canal
7. Intervertebral foramen
8. Annulus fibrosus
9. Nucleus pulposus
10. Intervertebral disc

Comments

Anatomical: The six ligaments are the intertransverse, the anterior longitudinal, the posterior longitudinal, the supraspinous, the interspinous and the ligamentum flavum. An intervertebral disc, made up of an annulus fibrosus and a nucleus pulposus, separates the two adjacent vertebrae. The thickness of the discs increases from the top to the bottom of the spinal column. The intervertebral foramen is a hole lying between the vertebral pedicles that allows the passage of spinal nerves, blood vessels and lymphatics.

Physiological: The ligaments keep the vertebrae and the intervertebral discs in place. They also help in absorbing shocks and making the column flexible.

Clinical: Lumbago is related to damage to the intervertebral disc at lumbar level resulting mostly from carrying heavy weights. It is a pain localised over the disc, without further spread. When the intervertebral disc is crushed, it can cause compression of a nerve root with pain in the thigh if L2, L3 or L4 is involved; compression of L5 or S1 causes sciatica.

The thoracic cage, anterior view

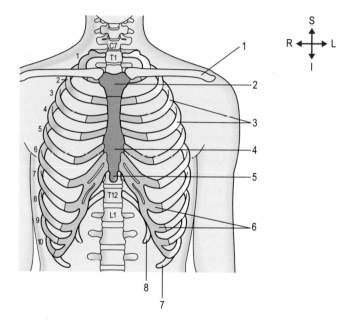

Fig 204

1. Clavicle
2. Manubrium sterni
3. Ribs
4. Body of sternum
5. Xiphoid process of sternum
6. Costal cartilages
7. Eleventh rib
8. Twelfth rib

Comments

Anatomical: The thoracic cage is linked to the clavicles, the scapulae and the cervical vertebral column in its upper part and to the lumbar vertebral column in its lower part. The bones of the thoracic cage include the sternum, twelve pairs of ribs and twelve vertebrae. The sternum, which is the flat bone of the chest, is made up of the manubrium sterni, which articulates with the clavicles, of a body attached to the ribs and the pointed xiphoid process, which gives attachment to the diaphragm and the muscles of the abdominal wall. Costal cartilages attach the ribs to the sternum.

Physiological: The thoracic cage protects and keeps the lungs, the heart, the oesophagus, the viscera, the trachea and the lymph nodes in place. It is flexible because of the arrangement of the ribs and the presence of cartilage and the intercostal muscles, and it moves with breathing.

Clinical: Pain, difficulty in breathing and even respiratory distress are suggestive of trauma to the ribs. The clinical diagnosis is geared to identifying the symptoms of respiratory, cardiovascular and neurological failure.

The sternum and its attachments, anterior view

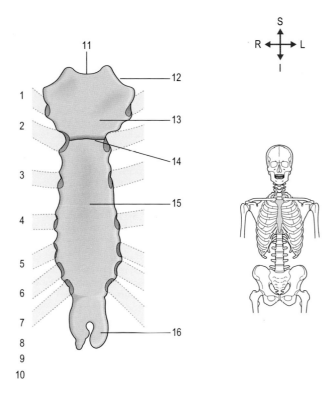

Fig 205

1 to 10. Ribs
11. Jugular (sternal) notch
12. Clavicular notch
13. Manubrium
14. Sternal angle
15. Body
16. Xiphoid process

Comments

Anatomical: The sternum, the flat bone located in the middle of the anterior aspect of the chest, is made up of spongy and compact bone. Its upper part is the manubrium, which articulates with the clavicles to form the sternoclavicular joints, and with the first two pairs of ribs. It has a jugular notch on its upper margin, and it has a sternal angle. The ribs are attached by the costal cartilages to its body or midsection. In its lower part, the xiphoid process gives attachment to the diaphragm and the muscles of the abdominal wall.

Physiological: The sternum provides attachment for the sternocleidomastoid muscle. Its bone marrow produces blood cells.

Clinical: The sternum can be felt under the skin. Because it contains spongy bone, it can be used to sample the bone marrow (via a sternal puncture).

A typical rib, seen from below

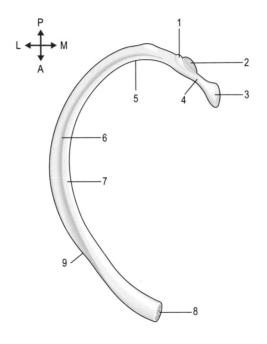

Fig 206

1. Tubercle
2. Articular facet for the transverse process
3. Head articulating with the vertebral body
4. Neck
5. Angle
6. Costal groove
7. Body
8. Depression for the costal cartilage
9. Inferior border

Comments

Anatomical: A rib is a long curved bone that articulates posteriorly with the vertebral column via a synovial joint. The first seven ribs articulate directly with the sternum and the other three indirectly, whereas the remaining two ribs are floating, with unattached ends. The ribs form joints between their tubercles and the transverse processes of the corresponding vertebrae.

Physiological: Contraction of the intercostal muscles allows the ribs to move during breathing. The costal groove provides passage to the intercostal nerves and blood vessels

Clinical: A fractured rib causes severe pain lasting for 1 or more months that is triggered by breathing movements, especially deep inspiration. Trauma to the lung can be a complication.

The right clavicle, seen from above

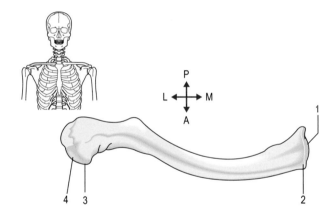

Fig 207

1. Articular facet for the sternum
2. Sternal end (medial)
3. Acromial end (lateral)
4. Articular facet for the scapula

Comments

Anatomical: The clavicle is an S-shaped long bone that attaches the upper limb to the axial skeleton. It has two articular facets, one for the scapula and the other for the sternum.

Physiological: The clavicle takes part in two joints, the sternoclavicular joint with the manubrium sterni and the acromioclavicular joint with the acromion of the scapula. Its deltoid tubercle corresponds to the site of insertion of the deltoid muscle.

Clinical: A fracture of the clavicle causes constant pain on movement of the upper limb, thus preventing its use. As a result, the patient's shoulder droops, the arm is stuck to the body and the hand supports the forearm.

The right scapula, posterior view

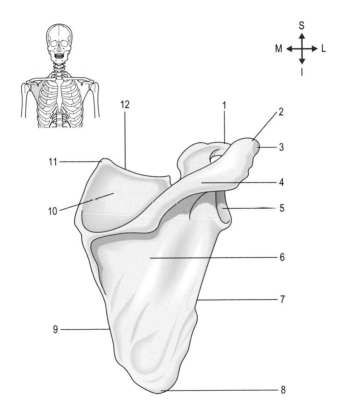

S
M ← → L
I

12 1 2
3
11
4
10
5

6

7

9

8

Fig 208

1. Coracoid process
2. Acromion
3. Articular facet for the clavicle
4. Spine
5. Glenoid cavity
6. Infraspinous fossa
7. Lateral border
8. Inferior angle
9. Medial border
10. Supraspinous fossa
11. Superior angle
12. Superior border

Comments

Anatomical: The triangular scapula is a flat bone in the thoracic wall. It has a concave glenoid cavity, which articulates with the head of the humerus to form the shoulder joint. The acromion is the spinous process that overhangs the shoulder. The muscles mobilising the shoulder joint are attached to the coracoid process.

Physiological: Because of its synovial nature, the acromioclavicular joint allows the shoulder girdle to be mobilised and thus increases its movements. The ligament and muscles maintain the stability of the shoulder joint.

Clinical: The wider the range of motion at a joint, the greater the risk of instability. A reduction in the range of movement at the shoulder joint can be due to a traumatic lesion (dislocation or fracture) or a neurological lesion.

The right humerus, anterior view

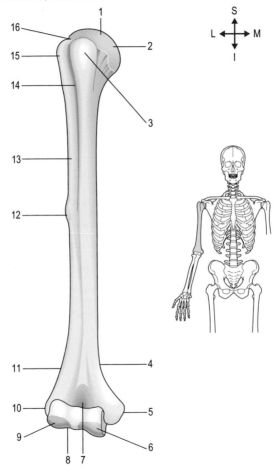

S
L ↔ M
I

Fig 209

1. Head
2. Articular facet for the glenoid cavity of the scapula
3. Lesser tubercle
4. Medial supracondylar ridge
5. Medial epicondyle
6. Articular facet for the ulna
7. Coronoid fossa
8. Trochlea
9. Capitulum with articular facet for the radius
10. Lateral epicondyle
11. Lateral supracondylar ridge
12. Deltoid tuberosity
13. Diaphysis (shaft)
14. Bicipital groove
15. Greater tubercle
16. Neck

Comments

Anatomical: The humerus, a bone of the upper limb, has two ends — the proximal end contains the head, the neck and two tubercles; the distal end, also called the condylar end, contains the trochlea and two epicondyles. The capitulum lies at the distal end of the humerus. The muscles are attached to its diaphysis (shaft). Between its two tubercles, the greater and the lesser, lies the bicipital groove, or intertuberous sulcus, which lodges the long head of the biceps. Its head articulates with the glenoid cavity of the scapula. The rotator cuff, made up of a combination of tendons and muscles, is inserted around the humeral head and covers it, thus reinforcing the capsule of the joint.

Physiological: The articular surfaces of the humerus, which are in contact with the ulna and the radius, allow the elbow to move. The trochlea articulates with the ulna and the capitulum articulates with the radius. The rotator cuff allows the arm to be extended and rotated. The humerus receives its blood supply from the humeral artery and its nerve supply from the radial and ulnar nerves.

Clinical: In case of fracture of the humerus, signs of damage to blood vessels and nerves must be looked for because of the proximity of these structures. Loss of function of the shoulder can be due to a lesion of the rotator cuff.

The right radius and ulna with the interosseous membrane, anterior view

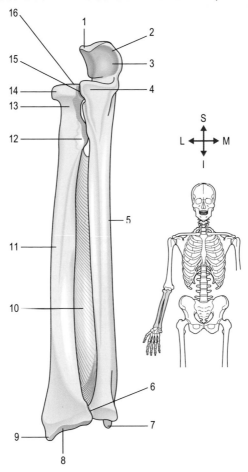

Fig 210

1. Olecranon
2. Articular facet for the trochlea of the humerus
3. Trochlear notch
4. Coronoid process
5. Shaft of ulna
6. Distal radioulnar joint
7. Styloid process of ulna
8. Articular facet for the scaphoid and lunate bones
9. Styloid process of radius
10. Interosseous membrane
11. Shaft of radius
12. Radial tuberosity
13. Neck of radius
14. Head of radius
15. Proximal radioulnar joint
16. Articular facet for the capitulum of the humerus

Comments

Anatomical: The ulna and the radius are the two bones of the upper arm, with the radius being the shorter. With the humerus, they form the elbow joint and, with the carpal bones, they form the wrist joint. They articulate with each other at the proximal and distal radioulnar joints. They are also attached to each other by a fibrous interosseous membrane, which maintains their relative positions regardless of the forces exerted on them by the elbow or the wrist. Both bones provide attachment to muscles.

Physiological: The radioulnar joints allow movements of flexion, pronation and supination. The radius allows flexion of the forearm, flexion and extension of the wrist, pronation (moving the palm of the hand to face upwards) and supination (moving the palm of the hand to face downwards). The ulna participates in the movement of rotation and of flexion and extension of the forearm on the upper arm and of pronation and supination of the forearm.

Clinical: The bones lie parallel to each other when the palm of the hand faces forwards.

The bones of the right hand, wrist and fingers, anterior view

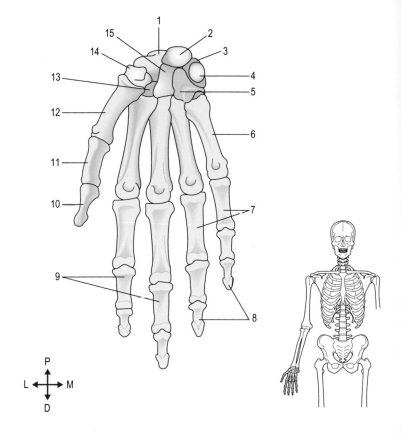

Fig 211

1. Scaphoid
2. Lunate
3. Triquetrum
4. Pisiform
5. Hamate
6. Fifth metacarpal
7. Proximal phalanges
8. Distal phalanges
9. Middle phalanges
10. Distal phalanx
11. Proximal phalanx
12. First metacarpal
13. Trapezoid
14. Trapezium
15. Capitate

Comments

Anatomical: The bones of the hand, the wrist and the fingers are, respectively, the five metacarpal bones, the eight carpal bones arranged in two rows of four each, and the 14 phalanges, (two for each thumb and three for each of the other fingers). The metacarpals, numbered from the thumb to the fifth metacarpal, lie between the carpal bones and the phalanges. The carpal bones are called the *scaphoid*, the *lunate*, the *triquetrum*, the *pisiform* (in the proximal row) and the *capitate*, the *trapezium*, the *trapezoid* and the *hamate* (in the distal row). These bones are linked to each other and kept in place by ligaments that allow them to move. The phalanges, two in the thumb and three in the other fingers, articulate with the metacarpals.

Physiological: The bones of the proximal row form part of the wrist joint. The hand is the organ of prehension. Its blood supply relies on the radial and ulnar arteries and veins, and its nerves come from the ulnar, median and radial nerves.

Clinical: In right-handed people, the right hand is more agile than the left, with the opposite seen in left-handed people. Those who are ambidextrous are able to use both hands with equal ease. Fractures of the scaphoid and dislocation of the lunate are common. Rheumatic diseases, in particular rheumatoid arthritis, often involve the wrist and the hand.

The right hip bone, lateral view

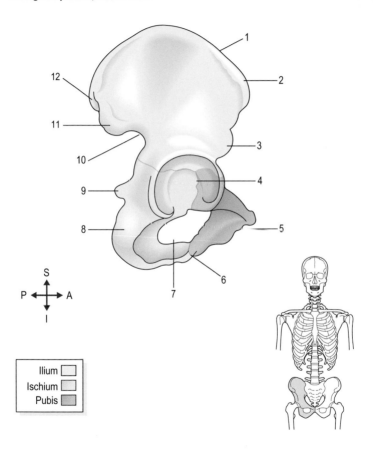

S
P ←→ A
I

Ilium ☐
Ischium ☐
Pubis ☐

Fig 212

1. Iliac crest
2. Anterior superior iliac spine
3. Anterior inferior iliac spine
4. Acetabulum, with lines indicating the sutures
5. Pubic symphysis
6. Union of ischium and pubis
7. Obturator foramen
8. Ischial tuberosity
9. Ischial spine
10. Greater sciatic notch
11. Posterior inferior iliac spine
12. Posterior superior iliac spine

Comments

Anatomical: The hip bone is made up of three fused bones — the ilium, the ischium and the pubis. It articulates with the femoral head to form the hip joint at the acetabulum, where these bones become fused.

Physiological: The ischial tuberosities and the sacroiliac joints act together to absorb the weight of the body and transfer it from the trunk to the lower limbs.

Clinical: During pregnancy and labour, the pubic symphysis becomes functionally looser. It can also be involved in chondrocalcinosis, which is an arthritic condition that is related to the deposition of microcrystals.

The components of the hip bone and the upper part of the left femur

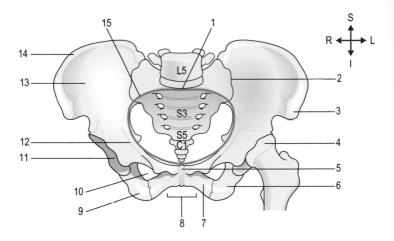

S
R ← → L
I

L5
S3
S5
C1

14
13
12
11
10
9

15
1
2
3
4
5
6

8   7

Fig 213

1. Sacral promontory
2. Sacroiliac joint
3. Anterior superior iliac spine
4. Head of femur
5. Pubic symphysis
6. Ischium
7. Pubis
8. Pubic arch
9. Ischial tuberosity
10. Obturator foramen
11. Acetabulum
12. Iliopectineal line
13. Ilium
14. Iliac crest
15. Pelvic inlet (superior pelvic aperture)

Comments

Anatomical: The pelvis is formed by the two hip bones, the sacrum and the coccyx. It is divided into two parts by the pelvic inlet or the superior pelvic aperture, which is made up of the sacral promontory and the iliopectineal line.

Physiological: The pelvis supports part of the weight of the body. With its shape and larger size and its light constituent bones, the female pelvis allows for passage of the baby during labour.

Clinical: Osteoarthritis of the hip is due to a shrinkage of the joint space between the femur and the hip bone. It causes hip pain of mechanical origin that starts with and is worsened by movement but is relieved by rest.

The left femur, seen from behind

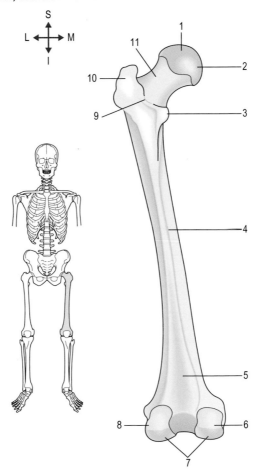

Fig 214

1. Articular facet for the acetabulum
2. Head
3. Lesser trochanter
4. Linea aspera
5. Popliteal surface
6. Medial condyle
7. Articular facets for tibia
8. Lateral condyle
9. Intertrochanteric line
10. Greater trochanter
11. Neck

Comments

Anatomical: The femur is the only bone in the thigh, the longest and heaviest bone in the body; it belongs to the lower limb. Its spherical head articulates with the hip bone to form the hip joint. The femoral neck is partly covered by the joint capsule. The two condyles at its distal end articulate with the tibia and the patella to form the knee joint.

Physiological: The femur transmits the weight of the body and can tolerate augmented levels of pressure during jumping.

Clinical: The signs and symptoms of fracture of the femoral neck include partial or total loss of the ability to move, distortion of the lower limb, with displacement of its axis, severe pain in the hip region exacerbated by palpation and possibly by swelling around the joint. Signs of vascular and neurological involvement must be watched for to spot the presence of damage to blood vessels and nerves, which can complicate the clinical picture.

The left tibia and left fibula with the interosseous membrane, anterior view

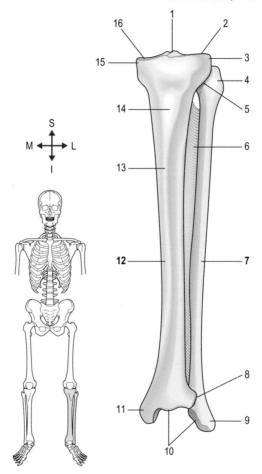

S
M ←→ L
I

Fig 215

1. Intercondylar eminence
2. Articular facet for the lateral femoral condyle
3. Lateral condyle
4. Head of fibula
5. Location of proximal tibiofibular joint
6. Interosseous membrane
7. Fibula
8. Location of distal tibiofibular joint
9. Lateral malleolus
10. Articular facets for talus
11. Medial malleolus
12. Tibia
13. Anterior border
14. Tibial tuberosity
15. Medial condyle
16. Articular facet for medial femoral condyle

Comments

Anatomical: The tibia, a leg bone, has two condyles that articulate with the femur to form the knee joint. It articulates with the head of the fibula to form the proximal tibiofibular joint, with the fibula to form the distal tibiofibular joint and with the talus and fibula to form the ankle joint. The medial malleolus is a prong-like extension of the tibia towards the ankle; the lateral malleolus is the distal end of the fibula, which is the thin bone of the leg. These are the facets that articulate with the talus.

Physiological: The fibula stabilises the ankle joint. The distal tibiofibular joint is weight-bearing and allows the body to be stable and mobile.

Clinical: The signs and symptoms of an ankle sprain include an acute pain, a sensation of something breaking, an immediate inability to use the ankle and an external swelling.

The bones of the left foot, seen from the side

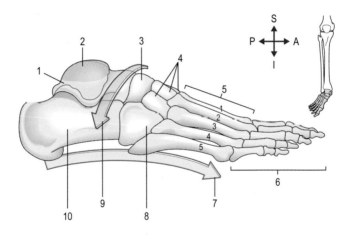

Fig 216

1. Talus
2. Articular facet for tibia
3. Navicular
4. Three cuneiforms
5. Five metatarsals
6. Fourteen phalanges
7. Longitudinal arch
8. Cuboid
9. Transverse arch
10. Calcaneus

Comments

Anatomical: The foot contains 26 bones. The five metatarsals form the dorsum of the foot and articulate with the tarsal bones and the phalanges; they are numbered from the inside to the outside of the foot. The seven tarsal bones that form the ankle are named the *talus*, the *calcaneus*, the *navicular*, the *cuboid* and the three *cuneiforms*. The calcaneus forms the heel, and the talus articulates with the tibia and the fibula to form the ankle joint. The 14 bones of the toes are the phalanges, two in the big toe and three in each of the others. The sole of the foot has a curved shape because of its constituent bones, ligaments and associated muscles. There are two arches — the longitudinal arch extending up from the heel to the toes and the transverse arch stretching across the foot.

Physiological: The foot bears the weight of the body in the standing position and allows locomotion to occur. The distal extremities of the metatarsals and the calcaneus allow the foot to rest on the ground. The foot is involved in balance, shock absorption and propulsion.

Clinical: The foot can have three different profiles, depending on the shape and orientation of the heads of the metatarsals. The tip of the big toe is the most distal in the Egyptian type of foot, the tip of the second toe is the most distal in the Greek type of foot, and the tips of the first three toes are at the same level distally in the Roman type of foot.

The tendons and ligaments supporting the arches of the left foot, medial view

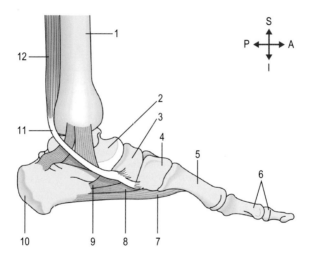

Fig 217

1. Tibia
2. Talus
3. Navicular
4. Medial cuneiform
5. First metatarsal
6. Phalanges
7. Long plantar ligament
8. Short plantar ligament
9. Spring ligament
10. Calcaneus
11. Posterior tibialis tendon
12. Posterior tibialis muscle

Comments

Anatomical: The curve of the foot from the heel to the toes is the longitudinal arch; the curve across the foot is the transverse arch.

Physiological: The arches of the foot allow the weight of the body to be evenly spread at rest or during movement. The numerous joints between the bones, the ligaments and the muscles allow the foot to remain elastic and stable at rest or during running or jumping. The tibialis posterior provides muscular support for the longitudinal arch. The short muscles, constituting the fleshy part of the foot, also help maintain the longitudinal arch. The plantar calcaneonavicular ligament acts as a spring (hence, the name *spring ligament*). The plantar ligaments support the longitudinal and the transverse arches. Inversion and eversion are, respectively, rotational movements of the sole of the foot as it moves medially or laterally.

Clinical: A normal footprint reflects the contact points of the longitudinal arch where the metacarpals and the calcaneus touch the ground, without involvement of the other bones. Pes planus (flat foot) arises when the longitudinal arch collapses, with recruitment of other bones for support; pes cavus (claw foot) arises when the arch becomes more concave.

A fibrous or fixed cranial joint

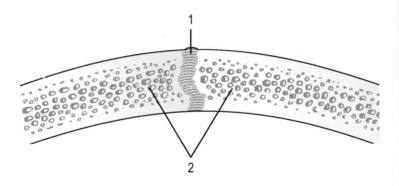

Fig 218

1. Fibrous joint
2. Bone

Comments

Anatomical: A fibrous joint often is the result of the junction of two bones by solid fibrous tissue.

Physiological: A fibrous joint often allows no movement to occur, as between the bones of the cranium. Some fibrous joints allow movement because of the flexibility provided by an interosseous membrane, as between the tibia and the fibula. The fibrous tissue then has two functions, to maintain the alignment of the bones and to provide some degree of flexibility.

Clinical: The cranial bones of a newborn are separated at birth by fibrous membranes, the fontanelles, which later become solid.

A cartilaginous joint between the bodies of adjacent vertebrae

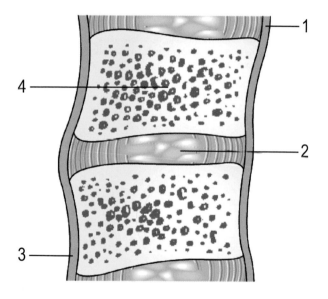

Fig 219

1. Ligament
2. Fibrocartilaginous disc (intervertebral disc)
3. Ligament
4. Vertebral body

Comments

Anatomical: A cartilaginous joint is a site of attachment between two bones, consisting of a cushion of shock-absorbing fibrocartilage.

Physiological: This cartilaginous joint can be mobilised or not and allows movements of the vertebrae to take place, depending on the presence of fibrocartilage, which can absorb shocks occurring between these two bones.

Clinical: The cartilaginous joints between the vertebrae C1 and L5, which have a fibrocartilaginous intervertebral disc, can be mobilised. The vertebrae of the coccyx and the sacrum are fused to each other and cannot be mobilised.

The basic structure of a synovial joint

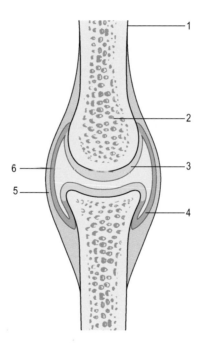

Fig 220

1. Periosteum
2. Bone
3. Articular cartilage
4. Synovial membrane
5. Capsule
6. Synovial cavity

Comments

Anatomical: A synovial joint is made up of hyaline articular cartilage, a capsule or capsular ligament, a synovial membrane and intracapsular and extracapsular structures. The ends of the bones are kept in place by a fibrous sheath. Its main feature is the presence of a capsule lubricated by a liquid that bathes the two articulating bones.

Physiological: Synovial joints are the most mobile of joints. Their movements include flexion, extension, abduction, adduction, circumduction, rotation, pronation, supination, inversion and eversion. The blood vessels and the nerves located near the joint supply the capsules and the muscles.

Clinical: Pain caused by movement and relieved by rest and the presence of an effusion of synovial fluid in the joint suggest some form of mechanical damage common in this type of joint, with the most likely cause being osteoarthritis. Other forms of arthritis of the inflammatory type are associated with pain that occurs at night, needs stretching exercises in the morning and improves with movement.

The right shoulder joint (1), cross section, seen from in front

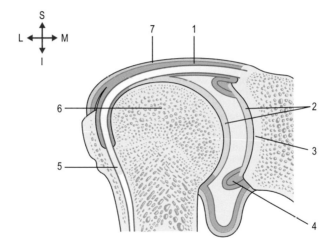

Fig 221

1. Synovial membrane
2. Articular cartilage
3. Glenoid cavity of the scapula
4. Glenoid labrum
5. Tendon of long head of the biceps
6. Head of the humerus
7. Capsular ligament

Comments

Anatomical: The shoulder joint is a synovial joint formed by the glenoid cavity of the scapula and the head of the humerus. Its synovial membrane, lying deep to the capsular ligament, surrounds the tendon of the long head of the biceps and the fibrocartilaginous glenoid labrum, which enlarges the glenoid cavity.

Physiological: This joint is very mobile, with movements of flexion, extension, abduction, adduction, lateral rotation, axial rotation and circumduction.

Clinical: Because of its great mobility, the shoulder joint has a high risk of dislocation, notably in children. A dislocation results in permanent displacement of the articular surfaces with respect to each other. The signs and symptoms of dislocation include pain on movement of the joint, the need to support the dislocated arm with the intact hand and distortion of the joint. The most serious complication is damage to the circumflex nerve.

The right shoulder joint (2), the supporting ligaments, seen from the front

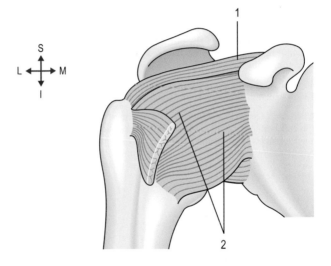

Fig 222

1. Coracohumeral ligament
2. Glenohumeral ligaments

Comments

Anatomical. The ligaments of the shoulder joint, which is a ball and socket joint, are the coracohumeral, the glenohumeral, the transverse humeral and the capsular ligaments.

Physiological: The coracohumeral, the glenohumeral and the transverse humeral ligaments keep the shoulder joint stable and in place. They are helped by muscles, particularly the muscles of the rotator cuff. The capsular ligament is loose and allows movements to occur.

Clinical: The shoulder joint is often dislocated. In cases of repeated dislocations associated with stretching of the tendons, it becomes unstable and may need surgical attention. A lesion of the rotator cuff causes severe pain in the shoulder and reduces joint mobility. It may take a long time to recover its mobility, ranging from a few months to a few years.

The right elbow and proximal radioulnar joints, cross section, seen from the front

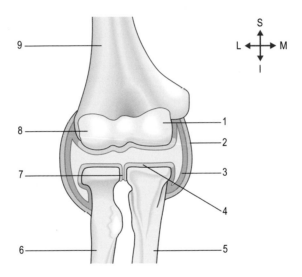

Fig 223

464

1. Trochlea
2. Capsular ligament
3. Synovial membrane
4. Articular cartilage
5. Ulna
6. Radius
7. Proximal radioulnar joint
8. Capitulum
9. Humerus

Comments

Anatomical: The elbow joint is a hinge joint formed by the articulation of three bones, the humerus (the trochlea and the capitulum), the ulna and the radius. The proximal radioulnar joint and the elbow joint are kept in place by a strong capsule and an extracapsular structure made up of anterior, posterior, medial and lateral ligaments. The capsular ligament covers the synovial membrane.

Physiological: There are only two movements, extension and flexion. The biceps and the brachialis are responsible for flexion of the forearm and the triceps is responsible for its extension.

Clinical: It is a very stable joint. A fracture at the elbow leads to misalignment, as occurs in all other joints. Its diagnostic features include pain in the arm, swelling and a visible distortion of the joint contour. The elbow is dislocated posteriorly. The complication to be avoided is a posttraumatic loss of mobility associated with incomplete extension of the elbow.

The proximal radioulnar joint, seen from above

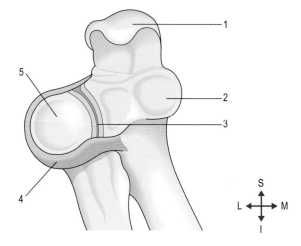

Fig 224

1. Olecranon
2. Ulna
3. Proximal radioulnar joint
4. Annular ligament
5. Radius

Comments

Anatomical: The proximal radioulnar joint is the articulation of the head of the radius with the radial notch of the ulna. It is surrounded by a strong capsule and a strong extracapsular ligament, the annular ligament.

Physiological: Its movements include pronation and supination. Pronation depends on the action of the pronator quadratus and the pronator teres and supination depends on the action of the biceps and the supinator muscle.

Section of the elbow joint, partially flexed, seen from the right side

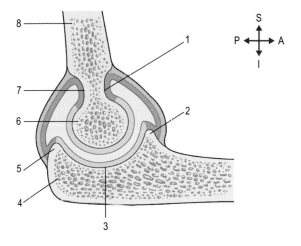

Fig 225

1. Coronoid fossa
2. Coronoid process
3. Trochlear notch
4. Ulna
5. Olecranon
6. Trochlea
7. Olecranon fossa
8. Humerus

Comments

Anatomical: At the upper end of the ulna, a hook-like cavity lodges the trochlea at the lower end of the humerus at an angle of 10 degrees anteriorly. The coronoid process of the ulna lies in the anterior aspect of the arm, near the proximal end of the ulna, in continuity with the olecranon.

Physiological: The movements at the elbow are flexion and extension and those at the proximal radioulnar joint are pronation and supination. The coronoid process maintains the stability of the elbow joint and prevents its dislocation.

The right wrist and distal radioulnar joint, cross section, seen from the front

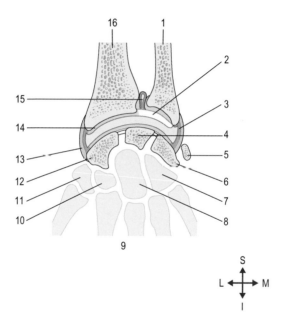

Fig 226

1. Ulna
2. Articular disc of white fibrocartilage
3. Synovial membrane
4. Lunate
5. Pisiform
6. Triquetrum
7. Hamate
8. Capitate
9. Proximal ends of the metacarpals
10. Trapezoid
11. Trapezium
12. Scaphoid
13. Capsular ligament
14. Articular cartilage
15. Distal radioulnar joint
16. Radius

Comments

Anatomical: The wrist (radiocarpal) joint is an ellipsoid joint formed by the radius, the scaphoid, the lunate and the triquetrum. The ulna is not part of the wrist joint. An articular disc of white fibrocartilage lies between the ulna and the cavity of the joint. The capsular ligament surrounds the synovial membrane.

Physiological: The movements at the wrist include flexion, extension, abduction and adduction.

Clinical: Fracture of the radius at the wrist (Colles' fracture) is common as a result of a fall onto the hand in older people or during sports. Pain on movement, swelling and loss of normal contours are the clinical findings.

The wrist and the distal radioulnar joint: their ligamentous support

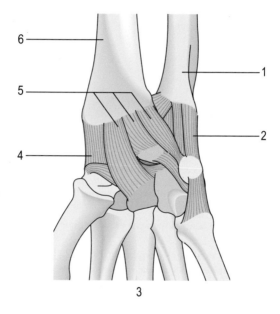

Fig 227

1. Ulna
2. Ulnar collateral ligament
3. Proximal ends of the metacarpal bones
4. Radial collateral ligament
5. Anterior radiocarpal ligament
6. Radius

Comments

Anatomical: The anterior, lateral and medial radiocarpal ligaments keep the wrist joint and the distal radioulnar joint in place.

Physiological: The movements of the wrist include flexion, extension, abduction (radial flexion), adduction (ulnar flexion) and circumduction. The ranges of flexion and adduction of the hand are greater than those of extension and abduction, respectively. Circumduction of the hand is the result of a combination of flexion, adduction, extension and abduction. The blood supply to the wrist depends on the palmar carpal arteries and veins, and its nerve supply comes from the radial, ulnar and medial nerves.

Clinical: Pain caused or exacerbated by movement and associated with swelling suggests a sprain of the wrist, with or without a ligamentous rupture. The risk for such an event is increased during a fall or a sports accident. In rheumatoid arthritis, the wrist and the joints of the hand are almost constantly painful.

The carpal tunnel and the synovial sheaths at the wrist and in the hand: right hand, palmar view

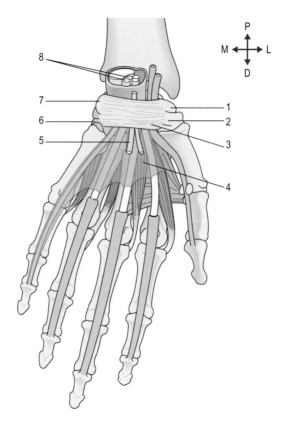

Fig 228 The sheaths are shown in *blue* and the tendons in *white*.

1. Scaphoid
2. Trapezium
3. Flexor retinaculum
4. Synovial sheath (in *blue*)
5. Median nerve
6. Hamate
7. Pisiform
8. Tendons of flexor muscles (in *white*)

Comments

Anatomical: The carpal tunnel is the space bounded by the distal row of carpal bones (the hamate and the trapezium) and in which the flexor retinaculum, the tendons of the flexor muscles of the fingers and the median nerve are lodged. The scaphoid and the pisiform belong to the proximal row of carpal bones. There are many synovial joints in the hand, and they are located between the constituent bones — for example, between the carpal bones, the carpal bones and the metacarpals, the metacarpals and the proximal phalanges. The movements of the fingers depend on tendons and not on muscles.

Physiological: The synovial fluid inside the synovial sheath prevents the tendons from rubbing against the bones. The movements of the fingers include flexion, extension, abduction, adduction and circumduction. The joints of the fingers, being of the hinge variety, allow only flexion and extension to occur. The area is supplied by the median nerve.

Clinical: The thumb is the most mobile finger because of its ellipsoid joints and can touch every other finger and the palm of the hand. Pain in the hand, paraesthesia and pins and needles in the fingers occurring at night, as well as loss of motor function, support the diagnosis of carpal tunnel syndrome, which affects mostly the first three fingers and is due to compression of the median nerve along its passage.

The left hip joint (1), anterior view

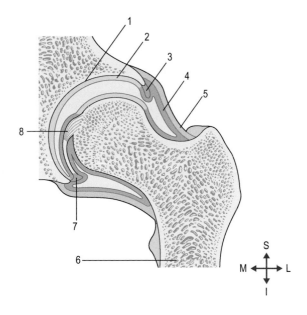

Fig 229

1. Acetabulum of the hip bone
2. Articular cartilage
3. Acetabular labrum
4. Synovial membrane
5. Capsular ligament
6. Femur
7. Acetabular labrum
8. Ligament of head of femur

Comments

Anatomical: The hip joint is a ball and socket joint between two bones, the hip bone and the femur. The capsular ligament covers most of the femoral head. The acetabular labrum is a fibrocartilaginous ring, attached to the hip bone and that delimits the articular cavity in the hip bone. The intraarticular ligament is the ligament of the head of the femur.

Physiological: The acetabular labrum plays a crucial role by controlling the range and types of movement in the joint — flexion, extension, abduction, adduction, rotation and circumduction — and maintaining its stability. This joint carries the full weight of the body in the standing position.

Clinical: Pain in the inguinal region on walking and difficulty in performing some movements of flexion and rotation suggest osteoarthritis of the hip joint. It is due to the natural course of ageing of the joint and is associated with progressive thinning of the articular cartilage, the distorting effect of direct contact between the exposed surfaces of the bones and, occasionally, the development of an intraarticular effusion.

The left hip joint (2), supporting ligaments

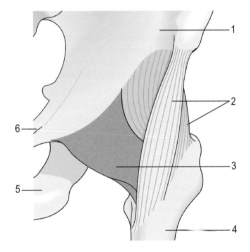

Fig 230

1. Ilium
2. Iliofemoral ligament
3. Pubofemoral ligament
4. Femur
5. Ischium
6. Pubis

Comments

Anatomical: The extraarticular ligaments of the hip joint are the iliofemoral, the pubofemoral and the ischiofemoral ligaments. Its intraarticular ligament is the ligament of the head of femur.

Physiological: The hip joint is kept in place by the ligaments and by the periarticular muscles.

Clinical: The signs and symptoms of hip dislocation include pain in the groin, distortion of the joint contour, abnormal orientation of the lower limb, asymmetry between the right and left hip joints and, possibly, some shortening of the affected limb. One must also look for secondary complications, such as a bone fracture, damage to the femoral artery and skin lacerations

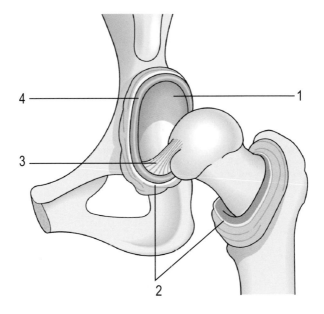

Fig 231 The femoral head and the acetabulum have been separated to show the acetabular labrum and the ligament of the head of femur.

1. Acetabulum
2. Capsular ligament (cut)
3. Ligament of the head of the femur
4. Acetabular labrum

Comments

Anatomical: The acetabular labrum is a fibrocartilaginous ring attached to the hip bone. It forms the rim of the acetabulum and deepens the cavity of the hip joint. The ligament of the head of femur lies inside the joint.

Physiological: The ligament of the head of femur helps maintain the stability of the joint.

Clinical: Rupture of the ligament of the head of femur can damage the accompanying artery and lead to necrosis of the femoral head.

The left knee joint (1), seen from in front

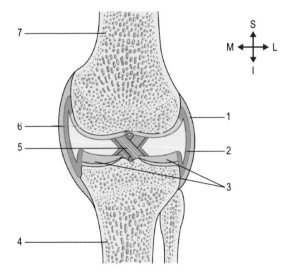

Fig 232

1. Capsular ligament
2. Synovial ligament
3. Menisci (semilunar cartilages)
4. Tibia
5. Cruciate ligament
6. Articular cartilage
7. Femur

Comments

Anatomical: The knee joint is a hinge joint made up of three articulating bones — the femur, the tibia and the patella. Because the femur and the tibia do not fit together perfectly, the space between them is filled by the semilunar cartilages or the menisci, which are mobile and malleable fibrocartilaginous discs that rest on the tibial condyles and the intraarticular fat pads. The synovial membrane does not coat the menisci but covers the cruciate ligaments, which cross each other and attach the femur to the tibia.

Physiological: The menisci bridge the gap between the femoral condyles and the tibial articular surface, stabilise and lubricate the joint and absorb the weight of the body and shocks. The periarticular muscles protect the joint. As a hinge joint, its movements are limited to flexion and extension. It can only move along one axis.

Clinical: When the shape of the menisci can adapt to the positions of the articulating bones during movements, the joint is stable. A pain on its own or that is associated with joint swelling suggests a meniscal lesion. Pain on movement made worse by a cracking sound, knee instability and a haemorrhagic effusion in the joint (haemarthrosis) suggest a severe sprain of the knee.

The left knee joint (2), the menisci and the cruciate ligaments

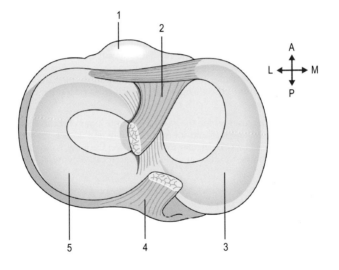

Fig 233

1. Tubercle
2. Anterior cruciate ligament
3. Medial meniscus
4. Posterior cruciate ligament
5. Lateral meniscus

Comments

Anatomical: There are two cruciate ligaments, one anterior and the other posterior. The medial and lateral menisci are mobile and malleable fibrocartilaginous discs on top of the tibial condyles. They are attached to the tibial intercondylar eminence.

Physiological: The menisci act as stabilisers, shock absorbers and distributors of stresses and lubricants by controlling the absorption and secretion of synovial fluid in the joint. The cruciate ligaments prevent forward displacement and excessive rotation in the joint. The periarticular ligaments support the joint. Being a hinge joint, it can perform only flexion and extension, with movements along only one axis.

Clinical: A rupture or tear of a cruciate ligament can be partial or complete and affect one or both of these ligaments in the same knee. The anterior cruciate is most often involved as a result of a sudden change of direction in running or jumping, for example.

The left ankle joint (1), anterior view

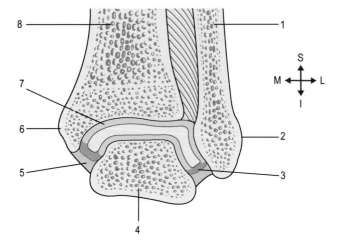

Fig 234

1. Fibula
2. Lateral malleolus
3. Synovial membrane
4. Talus
5. Capsular ligament
6. Medial malleolus
7. Articular cartilage
8. Tibia

Comments

Anatomical: The ankle joint is a hinge joint formed by the distal ends of the tibia and the fibula, the medial and lateral malleoli and the talus. It is held in place by the medial collateral ligament (the deltoid ligament) and the lateral collateral ligament.

Physiological: The ankle allows dorsiflexion and plantar flexion to take place. During dorsiflexion, the toes are raised towards the calf; during plantar flexion, the tips of the toes are extended. The tarsal bones allow inversion and eversion of the foot to occur. Foot inversion is the rotational movement that tilts the sole of the foot inwards; foot eversion tilts the sole of the foot outwards.

Clinical: Pain and difficulty in moving the joint are clinical indications of osteoarthritis.

The left ankle joint (2), supporting ligaments, medial view

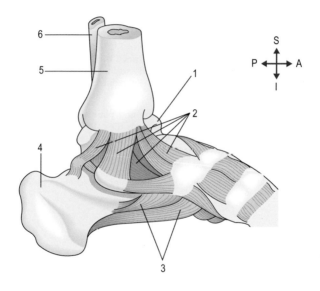

Fig 235

1. Talus
2. Components of the deltoid ligament
3. Plantar ligaments
4. Calcaneus
5. Tibia
6. Fibula

Comments

Anatomical: The ankle joint connects the distal ends of the tibia and fibula (the medial and lateral malleoli) and the talus. The lateral collateral ligament consists of a fan-like arrangement of three ligaments originating from the lateral malleolus at the distal end of the fibula. The medial collateral ligament (the deltoid), also fan-like, connects the medial malleolus to the talus and the calcaneus. The tendons of the leg muscles responsible for movements of the foot surround the ankle joint.

Physiological: The deltoid and the plantar ligaments support and stabilise the ankle joint, allowing it to bear the weight of the body.

Clinical: The most common lesion of the ankle is a sprain due to stretching of the lateral collateral ligament, caused by torsion of the inverted foot and ankle during a misstep or a bad landing after a jump. It gives rise to pain, which is exacerbated by movement of the joint and thus curtails its use. A swelling behind the ankle, along with the inability to stand on tiptoe, would suggest a rupture of the Achilles tendon, which can occur during quinolone antibiotic therapy.

The main muscles of the right side of the face, head and neck

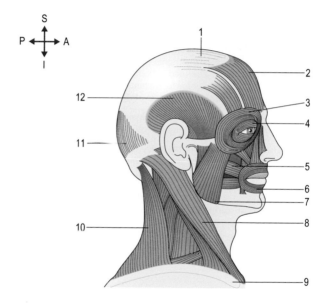

Fig 236

1. Epicranial aponeurosis
2. Occipitofrontalis (anterior part)
3. Orbicularis oculi
4. Levator palpebrae superioris
5. Buccinator
6. Orbicularis oris
7. Masseter
8. Sternocleidomastoid
9. Clavicle
10. Trapezius
11. Occipitofrontalis (posterior part)
12. Temporalis

Comments

Anatomical: There are many muscles of the face and neck, with the sternocleidomastoid and the trapezius belonging to the neck. The sternocleidomastoid is inserted into the temporal and occipital bones above and arises from the sternum and the clavicle below. The buccinator arises from the mandible and is inserted into the angle of the mouth. The occipitofrontalis arises from the epicranial aponeurosis. The orbicularis oris surrounds the mouth, and its fibres arise from the maxilla and the mandible.

Physiological: The temporalis pulls the mandible upwards and backwards and closes the mouth. The buccinator allows a person to blow, masticate and draw the angles of the mouth backwards and to the sides. The orbicularis oris allows a person to push the lips forward, close them, speak, whistle and masticate. The function of the masseter is mastication. The occipitofrontalis raises the eyebrows and helps express emotions. The levator palpebrae superioris elevates the upper eyelid, whereas the orbicularis oculi closes and protects the eye, maintains the drainage of tears and produces vertical wrinkles on the forehead. The trapezius raises and lowers the shoulders, pulls the shoulders and the head backwards and turns the head. The sternocleidomastoid allows the head to be flexed, inclined to the side and rotated.

Clinical: Torticollis (stiff neck) is an abnormal orientation of the head and neck that combines bending to one side and rotation of the head. The appearance of lateral wrinkles around the eyes is due to the loss of elasticity of the skin overlying the orbicularis oris.

The main muscles of the right side of the back

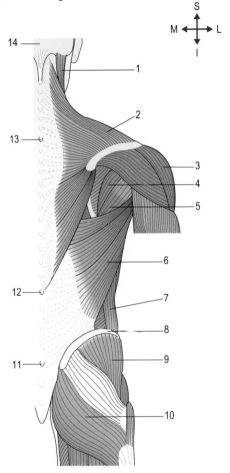

Fig 237

1. Sternocleidomastoid
2. Trapezius
3. Deltoid
4. Teres minor
5. Teres major
6. Latissimus dorsi
7. External oblique
8. Iliac crest
9. Gluteus medius
10. Gluteus maximus
11. Fifth lumbar vertebra (L5)
12. Twelfth thoracic vertebra (T12)
13. Seventh thoracic vertebra (T7)
14. Occiput

Comments

Anatomical: The muscles of the back are symmetrically arranged on either side of the vertebral column; they include the trapezius, latissimus dorsi, teres major, psoas, quadratus lumborum and erector spinae (sacrospinalis) muscle complex, which stretches from the sacrum to the occipital bone.

Physiological: The trapezius extends the head and elevates the shoulder, the teres major and the latissimus dorsi produce adduction, rotation and extension of the arm, the psoas produces flexion of the hip and the quadratus lumborum produces extension of the vertebral column, but ipsilateral flexion if the muscle contracts only on one side. The erector spinae produces extension of the vertebral column.

Clinical: Back pain can be due to muscle weakness secondary to excessive use, poor muscle function, bad posture, a sedentary lifestyle and a lack of exercise. Muscle pain must be distinguished from that associated with diseases of the spine, such as osteoarthritis, inflammatory arthritis and intervertebral disc herniation.

The muscles of the anterior abdominal wall

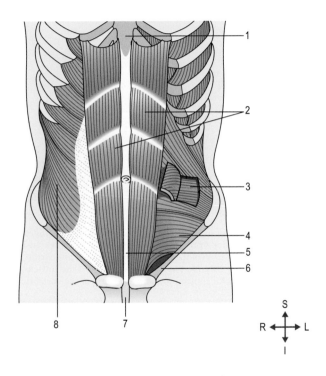

Fig 238

1. Sternum
2. Rectus abdominis muscles
3. Transversus abdominis (after reflection of the oblique muscles)
4. Internal oblique muscle (after removal of the external oblique)
5. Linea alba
6. Inguinal ligament
7. Pubic symphysis
8. External oblique muscle

Comments

Anatomical: The main muscles of the anterior abdominal wall are the rectus abdominis, the internal oblique, the external oblique and the transversus abdominis. The transversus, rectus and oblique muscles form the wall of the abdominal cavity, which contains the viscera. A median linea alba, which is a tendinous raphe, stretches from the xiphoid process of the sternum to the pubic symphysis.

Physiological: These muscles support the body, the abdomen, the vertebral column, the pelvis, and the thoracic cages and allow them to move. They participate in breathing, walking and weight-bearing. During expiration, the transversus contracts and raises the diaphragm towards the thoracic cage. The oblique muscles rotate and flex the trunk forwards and tilt the pelvis backwards. These muscles receive their nerve supply from the lower thoracic intercostal nerves.

Clinical: Weakening of the abdominal wall affecting the linea alba, the umbilicus and the inguinal canal can lead to herniation of the digestive organs, which sometimes requires surgical treatment.

The deep muscles of the posterior abdominal wall, anterior view

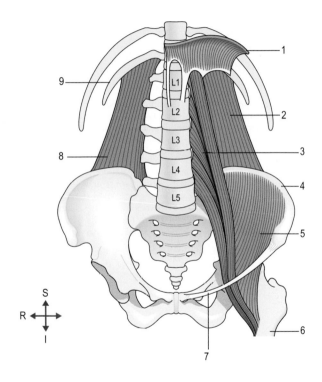

Fig 239

1. Diaphragm (cut)
2. Quadratus lumborum
3. Psoas major
4. Iliac crest
5. Iliacus
6. Femur
7. Inguinal ligament
8. Quadratus lumborum
9. Twelfth rib

Comments

Anatomical: The main muscles of the posterior abdominal wall are the psoas, running inferiorly and laterally, the iliacus, lying lateral to the inferior part of the psoas and the quadratus lumborum, running along the lumbar vertebrae and lying lateral to the superior part of the psoas. The inguinal ligament, stretching from the anterior superior iliac spine to the pubic tubercle, takes part in the formation of the inguinal canal, which runs obliquely across the abdominal wall and contains the round ligament in women and the spermatic cord in men.

Physiological: These muscles support the body, the abdomen, the vertebral column, the pelvis and the thoracic cage, and participate in their movements. They receive their nerve supply from branches of the lumbar plexus.

Clinical: Weakening of the abdominal wall at the level of the inguinal canal leads to an inguinal hernia. Posterior abdominal pain at the level of the iliacus and the psoas muscles can suggest disease of organs such as the kidney, the caecum, the appendix, the sigmoid colon and the pancreas or of nerves of the abdominal wall because of their proximity. Pain can be felt in the pubic region (pubalgia) by people engaged in sports, such as a footballer.

Transverse section of the muscles and aponeuroses of the anterior abdominal wall

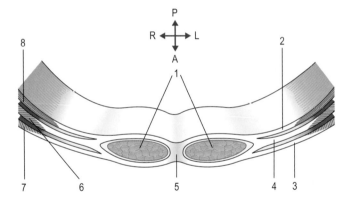

Fig 240

1. Recti abdominis
2. Aponeurosis of transverse abdominis
3. Aponeurosis of internal oblique
4. Aponeurosis of external oblique
5. Linea alba
6. Internal oblique muscle
7. External oblique muscle
8. Transversus abdominis muscle

Comments

Anatomical: The abdominal wall is divided lengthwise by the median linea alba, a tendinous raphe stretching from the sternal xiphoid process to the pubic symphysis. On either side of the abdominal wall, the muscles are symmetrical. They are the rectus abdominis, the internal oblique, the external oblique and the transversus abdominis muscles. These muscles are attached to one another by aponeuroses, which are bands of tendinous tissue that help keep the muscles together. The transversus, the rectus and the oblique muscles form the wall of the abdominal cavity, which contains the soft viscera.

Physiological: These muscles support the body, the abdomen, the vertebral column, the pelvis and the thoracic cage and allow them to move. They participate in breathing, walking and weight-bearing. They are supplied by the lower thoracic intercostal nerves.

Clinical: With age, the muscles of the abdominal wall become weaker, which can lead to an epigastric hernia through the linea alba.

The pelvic floor muscles in women

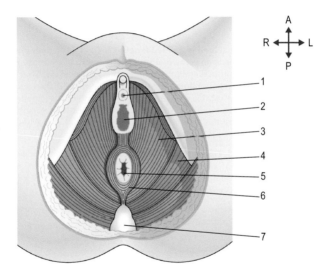

Fig 241

1. Urethral orifice
2. Vaginal orifice
3. Levator ani
4. Ischiococcygeus
5. Anal orifice
6. External anal sphincter
7. Coccyx

Comments

Anatomical: The muscles forming the pelvic floor stretch from the pubic bone to the coccyx. The levator ani is a flat muscle supplied by a terminal branch of the pudendal nerve. The ischiococcygeus is a thin muscle, which is buried deep in the pelvis and forms the dorsal part of the pelvic floor.

Physiological: The pelvic floor muscles support the pelvic organs—the uterus, the bladder and the intestine—and act as sphincters. They maintain continence by exerting pressure during micturition and defaecation. The levator ani elevates the anus and narrows the pudendal cleft. It also acts as a sphincter by bolstering the muscular tone of the pelvic floor.

Clinical: In men, these muscles support the bladder and the intestine. The muscles of the pelvic floor can be weakened by pregnancy, childbirth, a surgical operation on the prostate or old age. Weakening of the muscles of the pelvic floor can lead to urinary incontinence and prolapse of the genital organs. They can be strengthened by performing pelvic floor exercises.

The main muscles that mobilise the joints of the upper limb (1), anterior view

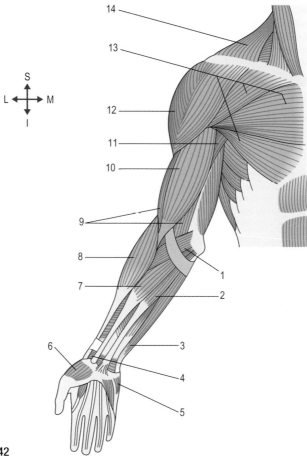

Fig 242

1. Pronator teres
2. Palmaris longus
3. Flexor carpi ulnaris
4. Pronator quadratus
5. Hypothenar muscles
6. Thenar muscles
7. Flexor carpi radialis

8. Brachioradialis
9. Brachialis
10. Biceps brachii
11. Coracobrachialis
12. Deltoid
13. Pectoralis major
14. Trapezius

Comments

Anatomical: There are many muscles that mobilise the shoulder and the upper limb, including the deltoid, pectoralis major, coracobrachialis, biceps, brachialis, triceps, pronator quadratus, brachioradialis, pronator teres, supinator, flexor carpi radialis, flexor carpi ulnaris, extensor carpi radialis brevis, extensor carpi radialis longus, palmaris longus, extensors of the fingers and the muscles that control the movements of the fingers. The thenar muscles are located in the lateral part of the hand and comprise the short muscles of the thumb.

Physiological: The role of these muscles is to stabilise the union between the bones of the axial skeleton and those of the upper limb. The pectoralis major flexes and adducts the arm; the biceps flexes and stabilises the shoulder, supinates the arm and flexes the elbow. The brachialis flexes the wrist; the coracobrachialis flexes the arm at the shoulder. The brachioradialis flexes the elbow and supinates the arm; the pronator teres pronates the forearm and flexes the elbow. The pronator quadratus allows pronation to occur and stabilises the radioulnar joint. The thenar muscles abduct, adduct and flex the thumb. The hypothenar muscles abduct and flex the little finger.

Clinical: Amyotrophic lateral sclerosis is due to a degeneration of the motor neurones, leading to a progressive weakening and eventually to paralysis of all the muscles, including the respiratory muscles. The muscles of the hand are affected early, especially those of the first interosseous space, whose atrophy is suggestive of amyotrophic lateral sclerosis if associated with cramps and muscle twitches.

The main muscles that mobilise the joints of the upper limb (2), posterior view

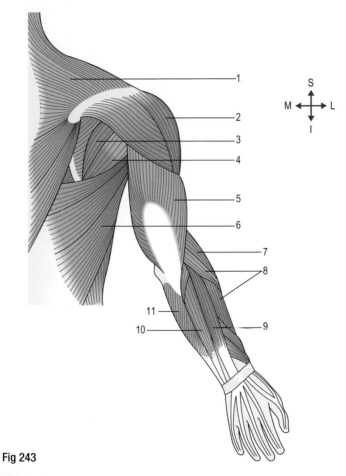

Fig 243

1. Trapezius
2. Deltoid
3. Teres minor
4. Teres major
5. Triceps
6. Latissimus dorsi
7. Brachioradialis
8. Extensors carpi radialis (brevis and longus)
9. Extensor digitorum
10. Extensor carpi ulnaris
11. Flexor carpi ulnaris

Comments

Anatomical: There are many muscles that mobilise the joints of the shoulder and the upper limb, including the deltoid, the pectoralis major, the coracobrachialis, the biceps, the brachialis, the triceps, the pronator quadratus, the brachioradialis, the pronator teres, the supinator, the flexor carpi radialis, the flexor carpi ulnaris, the extensor carpi radialis brevis, the extensor carpi radialis longus, the palmaris longus, the extensor muscles of the fingers and the muscles controlling the movements of the fingers.

Physiological: These muscles stabilise the union between the bones of the axial skeleton and those of the upper limbs; they also stabilise the movements of the shoulders and of the upper limbs. The deltoid flexes, abducts and extends the shoulder, the latissimus dorsi adducts, flexes and medially rotates the arm, the teres minor laterally rotates the arm. The teres major adducts and medially rotates the arm. The brachioradialis flexes the elbow and supinates the arm; the triceps extends the elbow.

The main muscles of the left lower limb (1), anterior view

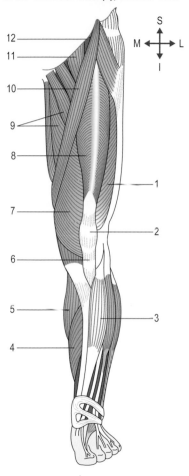

Fig 244

1. Vastus lateralis
2. Patellar region
3. Tibialis anterior
4. Soleus
5. Gastrocnemius
6. Patellar ligament (quadriceps tendon)
7. Vastus medialis
8. Rectus femoris
9. Hip adductors
10. Sartorius
11. Psoas
12. Iliacus

Comment

Anatomical: The muscles of the hip and of the lower limb include the psoas, the iliacus, the quadriceps femoris, the obturator muscles, the glutei, the sartorius, the adductors, the hamstrings, the gastrocnemius, the tibialis anterior and the soleus.

Physiological: These muscles carry the weight of the body, distribute it equally during walking or running, absorb shocks and allow the body to move. Many muscles participate in the movements of flexion that take place at a joint. The psoas, the iliacus, the quadriceps and the rectus femoris are responsible for hip flexion, the obturators are responsible for rotation at the hip, the adductors are responsible for adduction and medial rotation, the sartorius is responsible for flexion and abduction at the hip and for knee flexion, the gastrocnemius is responsible for flexion of the hip and the ankle, the tibialis anterior is responsible for dorsiflexion of the foot and the soleus is responsible for flexion of the ankle.

Clinical: Flexibility and mobility decline with age because of the stiffening effects of degenerative changes in the cartilage and connective tissue.

The main muscles of the left lower limb (2), posterior view

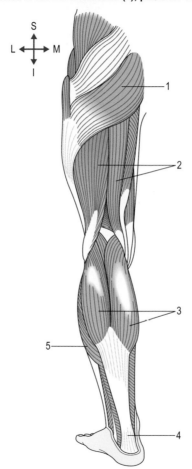

Fig 245

1. Glutei
2. Hamstrings
3. Gastrocnemius
4. Calcaneal (Achilles) tendon
5. Soleus

Comments

Anatomical: The glutei, the hamstrings, the gastrocnemius and the soleus are the other main muscles of the lower limb.

Physiological: They allow the lower limb to move. The glutei are responsible for extension, abduction and rotation at the hip, the hamstrings are responsible for knee flexion, the gastrocnemius is responsible for knee and ankle flexion and the soleus is responsible for ankle flexion.

The reproductive system

The female external genitalia

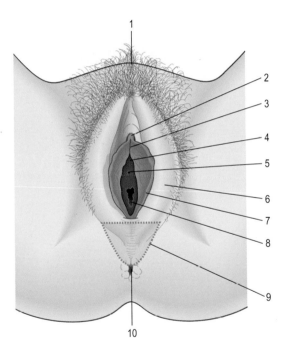

Fig 246

1. Mons pubis
2. Clitoris
3. Frenulum of clitoris
4. Vestibule
5. External urethral orifice
6. Labium majus
7. Labium minus
8. Vaginal orifice
9. Perineal region
10. Anus

Comments

Anatomical: The female external genitalia consist of the labia majora, the labia minora, the clitoris, the vaginal orifice, the vestibule, the hymen and the vestibular glands (Bartholin's glands). The perineum is the triangular area, with the labia minora forming its base and the anal canal forming its apex.

Physiological: They receive their nerve supply from the pudendal nerve and their blood supply from the internal and external pudendal arteries, and they drain via a venous plexus into the external iliac veins. The lymphatics drain into the inguinal lymph nodes. The labia majora and the labia minora, which are folds of the skin, contain sebaceous and sweat glands. The clitoris has nerve endings and erectile tissue.

Clinical: The signs and symptoms of vulvovaginal candidiasis (a yeast infection) are redness, swelling and itching of the external genitalia, whitish or smelly discharge, pain in the vulva and vagina during sexual intercourse and a burning sensation during urination. Itching, a burning sensation and genital sores are suggestive of a herpes simplex infection.

Lateral view of the intrapelvic female genitalia and related structures

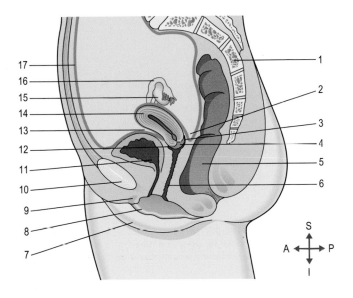

17

16

15

14

13

12

11

10

9

8

7

1

2

3

4

5

6

S

A ←→ P

I

Fig 247

1. Sacrum
2. Pouch of Douglas (rectouterine cul-de-sac)
3. Posterior vaginal fornix
4. Cervix
5. Rectum
6. Vagina
7. Labium majus
8. Labium minus
9. Clitoris
10. Pubic bone
11. Bladder
12. Anterior vaginal fornix
13. Vesicouterine pouch
14. Uterus
15. Ovary
16. Fallopian tube
17. Peritoneum

Comments

Anatomical: The vagina is a tube made up of three tissue layers—areolar tissue, a muscular coat and a stratified squamous epithelium with ridges and folds. It lies between the bladder and the anus, and it opens into the vestibule and the uterine cervix. The uterus is a hollow muscular organ that lies between the bladder and the rectum. The uterine cervix opens into the vagina at the external os. The hymen is a thin fold of mucous membrane that partially obstructs the vaginal orifice.

Physiological: The vagina acts as a receptacle during intercourse and provides a passage for the fetus during labour. The hymen, which does not entirely close the vaginal orifice, allows the egress of menstrual blood.

Clinical: The axis of the uterus, running in an anterosuperior direction, is set obliquely at an angle of about 45 degrees. It can be anteverted, leaning forward and oriented anterosuperiorly as a whole, or anteflexed, tilting forward along its long axis. It is more often in the anteverted position. The hymen is stretched during sexual intercourse.

The intrapelvic female genitalia

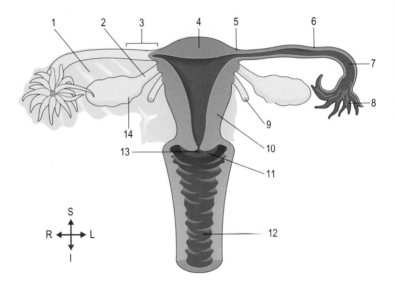

Fig 248

1. Broad ligament
2. Ovarian ligament
3. Isthmus
4. Uterine fundus
5. Intramural part of fallopian tube
6. Fallopian tube
7. Ampulla
8. Infundibulum with its fimbriae
9. Round ligament
10. Body of uterus
11. Cervix uteri
12. Vagina with folds
13. External os of cervix
14. Ovary

Comments

Anatomical: The female reproductive organs—the vagina, the uterus, the two fallopian tubes and the two ovaries—lie inside the pelvic cavity. The vagina is made up of three tissue layers, with the inner layer consisting of a squamous epithelium with transverse folds. The uterus has a body, a cervix and a fundus. The fallopian tubes, lying on either side of the uterus, are fimbriated at their distal extremities.

Physiological: The ovaries are the female gonads, which secrete the sex hormones and release the ova. The fallopian tubes transport the ovum from the ovary towards the uterus by peristaltic and ciliary activity. They are the sites of fertilisation of the ovum, which becomes the zygote, ready for migration into the uterus and for implantation.

Clinical: Secondary amenorrhoea is the absence of menstruation for over 3 months in a previously normally menstruating woman. It can also be primary when it occurs in young females who fail to menstruate. The duration of pregnancy is 40 weeks from the first day of the last menstrual period or 38 weeks from the last ovulation. An extrauterine pregnancy must be considered if menstruation is delayed and is associated with the passage of scanty, dark brown blood and pelvic pain.

The layers of the uterine wall

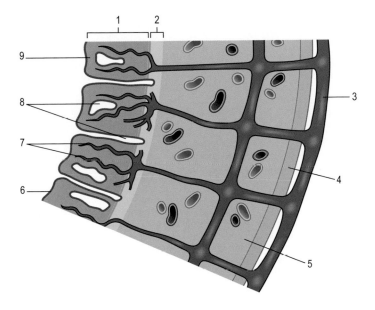

Fig 249 The green line shows the boundary between the functional and the basal layers of the endometrium.

1. Functional layer
2. Basal layer
3. Uterine artery
4. Perimetrium (serosa)
5. Myometrium
0. Columnar epithelium
7. Spiral arteries
8. Endometrial glands
9. Endometrium

Comments

Anatomical: The uterine wall is made up of three tissue layers—the perimetrium (serosa), the myometrium and the endometrium. The perimetrium consists of peritoneum that forms the vesicouterine and rectouterine cul-de-sacs. The broad ligament, made up of two layers of peritoneum, attaches the uterus to the pelvic wall. The myometrium is a muscle layer containing blood vessels and nerves. The endometrium consists of a columnar epithelium supported by connective tissue, which is richly supplied by the spiral arteries. The endometrium consists of two layers, a functional layer and a basal layer.

Physiological: The endometrium contains mucus-secreting glands. After puberty, its role is to receive and nourish the fertilised ovum. It undergoes changes during the menstrual cycle. The superficial layer of the endometrium—that is, the functional layer—thickens during the first part of the cycle and is then shed if there is no fertilised ovum. The basal layer allows the functional layer to regenerate for the next cycle.

Clinical: After puberty, the endometrium goes through a menstrual cycle that lasts about 28 days. Menstruation during the latter part of the cycle indicates a failure of fertilisation of an ovum; it can often be painful (dysmenorrhoea). Pain, abnormal bleeding, a sensation of heaviness and infertility are symptoms of endometrial dysfunction or of a uterine tumour (especially a benign leiomyoma). Dysmenorrhoea and infertility are the signs and symptoms of endometriosis (the presence of endometrium outside the uterine cavity), possibly due to the passage of the shed endometrium into the uterine tubes and the peritoneal cavity.

The main suspensory ligaments of the uterus

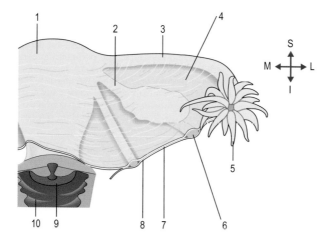

Fig 250

520

1. Uterus
2. Ovarian ligament
3. Fallopian tube
4. Peritoneum (broad ligament)
5. Fimbriated end of the fallopian tube
0. Suspensory ligament of the ovary
7. Cut border of the broad ligament
8. Round ligament
9. Uterine cervix
10. Vagina

Comments

Anatomical: The uterus is kept in place by its ligaments, the adjacent intrapelvic organs and the muscles of the pelvic floor. The broad, round, uterosacral, transverse cervical and pubocervical ligaments hold the uterus in place inside the pelvic cavity. The broad ligament is a double-layered fold of the peritoneum on either side of the uterus. The fibrous round ligament runs inside the broad ligament and is inserted into the labium majus.

Physiological: On both sides, the broad ligament attaches the ovary to the fallopian tube, with the help of the ovarian ligament.

Clinical: Infections of the tube (e.g., salpingitis), secondary to a sexually transmitted infection, can, if recurrent, cause progressive fibrosis of the tube, with tubal occlusion and infertility.

Section of an ovary showing the developmental stages of an ovarian follicle

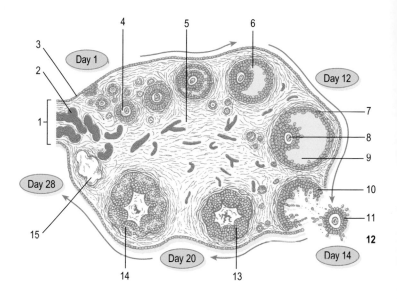

Fig 251

1. Mesovarium
2. Blood vessels
3. Germinal epithelium
4. Primordial follicle
5. Medulla
6. Maturing ovarian follicle
7. Mature ovarian follicle
8. Ovum
9. Follicular fluid
10. Ruptured follicle
11. Ovum
12. Ovulation
13. Formation of the corpus luteum
14. Fully formed corpus luteum
15. Corpus albicans

Comments

Anatomical: The ovary is made up of two tissue layers, the cortex and the medulla. The cortex surrounds the medulla and consists of connective tissue covered by the germinal epithelium. It contains the ovarian follicles, each of which harbours an ovum in various stages of maturation.

Physiological: Ovulation occurs once during the menstrual cycle in a woman's fertile period, with one mature follicle releasing an ovum into the fallopian tube. After ovulation, this follicle develops into a corpus luteum, which is replaced by fibrous tissue and becomes the scar-like corpus albicans on the ovarian surface.

Clinical: From birth, the connective tissue contains immature follicles. The fertilised ovum becomes the zygote, which will be implanted into the uterine wall to become first an embryo and then a fetus. The ovary can be the seat of benign tumours or cysts, especially in women between 20 and 25 years of age, as well as malignant tumours, which tend to be asymptomatic initially. Thus, they are diagnosed in their late stages, after they have spread into the pelvis and produced ascites.

The structure of the breast

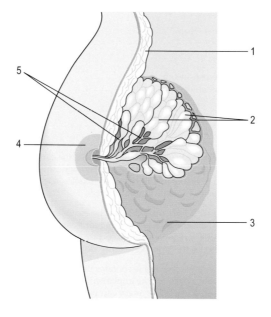

Fig 252

1. Adipose tissue
2. Lobules
3. Connective tissue
4. Areola surrounding the nipple
5. Lactiferous ducts

Comments

Anatomical: The breasts are two accessory glands in the female reproductive system. They consist of glandular, adipose and fibroconnective tissues. The breast is made up of lobes and lobules. The nipple is a projection of the breast and is surrounded by the pigmented areola, which contains many sebaceous glands.

Physiological: The glandular structures, or lobules of the breast, secrete milk, which is then carried to the nipple by the lactiferous ducts. The sebaceous glands of the areola lubricate the nipples during lactation. The breast is supplied by branches of the axillary, internal mammary and intercostal arteries and is drained by a circular periareolar venous plexus that drains into the mammary and axillary veins. Its lymphatics drain into the axillary lymph nodes. Its nerve supply comes from branches of the thoracic intercostal nerves.

Clinical: The breasts increase in size at puberty. After delivery, the secretion of milk is stimulated when the baby suckles. Any nipple discharge unrelated to pregnancy is abnormal. The signs and symptoms of breast cancer include the presence of a hard mass in the breast, a change in the skin of the breast (e.g., scaling, wrinkling, ulceration) and its size or contours, a unilateral nipple discharge, an inverted nipple and an indurated lymph node in the axilla.

The male reproductive organs and adjacent structures

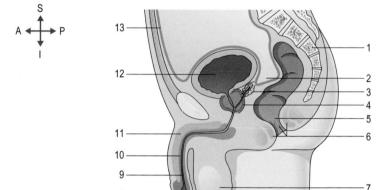

Fig 253

1. Sacrum
2. Retrovesical pouch
3. Seminal vesicle
4. Prostate
5. Rectum
6. Anal canal and anal sphincter
7. Scrotum containing the testes
8. Glans penis
9. Urethra
10. Corpus spongiosum
11. Corpus cavernosum
12. Bladder
13. Peritoneum

Comments

Anatomical: The male reproductive organs include the scrotum, the testes, the seminal vesicles, the ejaculatory ducts, the prostate, the urethra and the penis. The scrotum is a sac of pigmented skin overlying fibrous tissue and smooth muscle and is located below the pubic symphysis. The seminal vesicles are two fibromuscular reservoirs lying behind the prostate, close to the posterior wall of the bladder. The prostate is an accessory gland located behind the pubic symphysis, in front of the rectum and below the bladder, and flanked laterally by the levator ani muscles. It is traversed by the urethra and the ejaculatory ducts.

Physiological: The prostate is made up of a collection of small blind follicles that secrete prostatic fluid, which acts as a diluting fluid for the spermatozoa. The scrotum protects the testes, which are mixed glands with two functions: endocrine function, (androgen secretion) and exocrine function (spermatogenesis).

Clinical: Age, consumption of alcohol, smoking, and abnormalities in the formation, quality, quantity and movements of spermatozoa in the genital tract can be responsible for male subfertility. Aspermia is the complete absence of or presence of less than 0.5 mL of semen on ejaculation; azoospermia is the complete absence of spermatozoa in the ejaculate.

The testis: a section of the testis and its coats

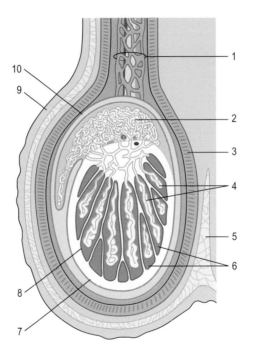

Fig 254

1. Spermatic cord
2. Epididymis
3. Smooth muscle
4. Seminiferous tubules
5. Septum of scrotum
6. Lobules
7. Tunica albuginea
8. Tunica vasculosa
9. Skin
10. Tunica vaginalis

Comments

Anatomical: The scrotum holds two testes, each of which is attached to a spermatic cord. Each testis is made up of 200 to 300 lobules filled with seminiferous tubules separated by interstitial Leydig cells. Each testis is invested with three coats — the tunica vaginalis, which is an external membrane derived from the abdominal and pelvic peritoneum; the tunica albuginea, which lies deep to the tunica vaginalis and contributes to the lobulation of the testis, and the tunica vasculosa, which contains the blood vessels embedded in connective tissue.

Physiological: The testes have two functions. They are the male reproductive organs responsible for spermatogenesis (the production of spermatozoa) from puberty onwards. The interstitial Leydig cells secrete testosterone, the primary male hormone responsible for the development of the genital organs. The luteinising hormone from the pituitary gland stimulates the Leydig cells to produce testosterone, which at puberty brings about the development of the secondary male sexual characteristics that transform boys into men.

Clinical: In embryos, the testes develop in the abdominal cavity, below the level of the kidneys and, by the 8th month of fetal life, they have descended into the scrotum and lost all contact with the abdominal cavity. During their descent into the scrotum, they carry some peritoneum, blood vessels, lymphatics, nerves and the vasa deferentia. Male puberty occurs at 10 to 14 years of age, with the following typical changes: increases in height and body weight; in hair growth on the face, in the axillae and on the thorax, the abdomen and the pubic region; in the size of the penis, scrotum and prostate; and in the size of the larynx, accompanied by a lowering of the voice, and in the thickness of the skin.

The testis: longitudinal section of the testis and the vas deferens

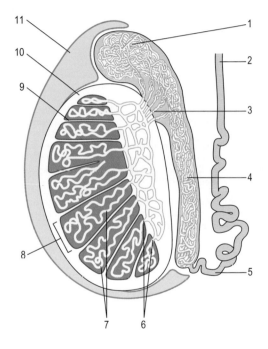

Fig 255

1. Head of epididymis
2. Vas deferens
3. Efferent ductules
4. Body of epididymis
5. Vas deferens
6. Straight seminiferous tubules
7. Coiled seminiferous tubules
8. Lobule
9. Testicular septum
10. Tunica albuginea
11. Tunica vaginalis

Comments

Anatomical: The epididymis is a long coiled organ connected to the testis that is made up of three parts—the head, the body and the tail. It is formed by the convergence of the seminiferous tubules and becomes the vas deferens in the spermatic cord as it leaves the scrotum.

Physiological: The spermatic cord supplies the testis with blood vessels and lymphatics. The seminiferous tubules produce the spermatozoa, which undergo maturation in the epididymis, where they are stored. Sperm production is stimulated by follicle-stimulating hormone, which comes from the pituitary.

Clinical: The production of a spermatozoon takes about 2 months, and almost 100 million spermatozoa are produced daily. Sperm production is under the influence of the intratesticular temperature, which is 3°C below the mean body temperature. The testes exhibit this temperature because of their location outside the abdominal cavity and the thinness of the scrotal wall that protects them. Failure of testicular descent into the scrotum, associated with a persistent intraabdominal location, is known as *cryptorchidism,* which can cause infertility if bilateral and increase the risk of testicular cancer.

Section of the prostate and associated reproductive structures

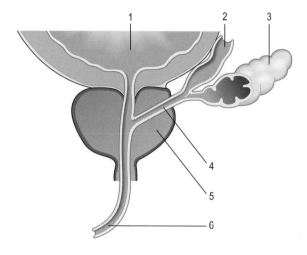

Fig 256

1. Bladder
2. Vas deferens
3. Seminal vesicle
4. Ejaculatory duct
5. Prostate
0. Urethra

Comments

Anatomical: The prostate is a gland located in the pelvic cavity that is anterior to the rectum and posterior to the pubic symphysis. It surrounds the urethra as it leaves the bladder. It is made up of blind glandular follicles that drain into their excretory ducts. The vas deferens measures about 45 cm and runs from the tail of the epididymis to the ejaculatory duct, which is formed by the fusion of the vas deferens with the duct of the ipsilateral seminal vesicle. The seminal vesicles are the fibromuscular reservoirs that lie posterior to the prostate, near the posterior wall of the bladder, and each vesicle opens into the ampulla of the corresponding vas deferens. Each ejaculatory duct, formed by the union of the vas deferens and the duct of the seminal vesicle, traverses the prostate to reach the prostatic urethra.

Physiological: The prostate produces a milky fluid, which constitutes 30% of the volume of semen and dilutes it for the spermatozoa. The seminal fluid is derived mostly from the seminal vesicles and from the prostate and Cowper's glands. At the moment of ejaculation from the urethra, the seminal vesicles release their stored seminal fluid; its abundant nutrient substances provide energy for the spermatozoa and protect them from the acidity of the vagina. The prostatic fluid contains a clotting enzyme that forms a coagulum for the spermatozoa in the vagina and promotes their transport towards the cervix uteri.

Clinical: The prostate normally weighs 8 g in young males and can weigh up to 40 g in later adult life because of benign prostatic hyperplasia. The seminal fluid is alkaline, with a pH between 7 and 8, and consists of vitamin C, vitamin B_{12}, prostaglandins, testosterone, sugars (sucrose and sorbitol) and electrolytes (magnesium, potassium and calcium). It makes up about 60% of the volume of semen.

The penis (1), seen from below

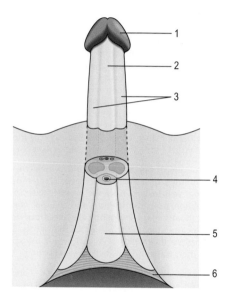

1
2
3
4
5
6

Fig 257

1. Glans penis
2. Corpus spongiosum
3. Corpus cavernosum
4. Urethra
5. Bulb of penis
6. Perineal membrane

Comments

Anatomical: The penis is anchored in the perineum at its root and is a mobile organ. It consists of erectile tissue, fibrous tissue and smooth muscle and has a very rich blood supply. Between the two columns of erectile tissue, the corpora cavernosa, lies the corpus spongiosum, made up of spongy tissue, which is also erectile. The bulbous extremity of the penis, the glans, contains the external urethral orifice (meatus); it is surrounded by a loose movable skin fold, the prepuce or foreskin. The urethra has three parts—the prostatic urethra from the bladder through the prostate, the membranous urethra from the prostate to the bulb of the penis and the spongy penile urethra passing through the corpora spongiosa to the urethral meatus.

Physiological: The penis receives somatic and autonomic nerves. It is supplied by branches of the internal pudendal artery and is drained by the internal pudendal veins on their way to the iliac veins. Parasympathetic stimulation causes active dilation of the penile arteries, with an increase in the flow of blood into the erectile tissues, followed by its retention due to passive obstruction of the venous outflow. The penis, when filled with blood, is then ready for coitus. It is the copulatory organ in males.

Clinical: During erection, the penis rises up in front of the abdomen, increases in volume and becomes hard. When flaccid, it looks like a cylinder flattened from front to back and hangs down in front of the scrotum.

The penis (2), seen from the side

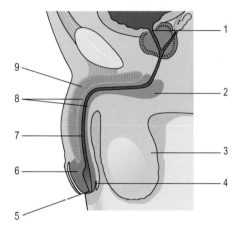

Fig 258

536

1. Internal urethral sphincter
2. Bulb of penis
3. Scrotum
4. Prepuce
5. External urethral sphincter
6. Glans penis
7. Urethra
8. Corpus spongiosum
9. Corpus cavernosum

Comments

Anatomical: The urethra has two sphincters, the internal sphincter at the level of the bladder neck above the prostate and the external sphincter that surrounds the spongy urethra.

Physiological: The male urethra acts as an excretory passage for urine and semen. Ejaculation or expulsion of sperm via the external urethral sphincter depends on the propulsive force elicited by sympathetic stimulation, with the help of semen-ejecting rhythmic contractions of the smooth muscle of the vas deferens, the walls of the seminal vesicles and the prostate. The latter two genital organs also contribute fluid to the semen.

Clinical: An ejaculate of semen of about 1.5 to 5 mL contains 40 to 80 million spermatozoa. Any abnormality in the ejaculate, such as haematospermia (blood in the semen) or a reduced force of ejaculation is clinically suggestive of some dysfunction of the genital system

Transverse section of the penis

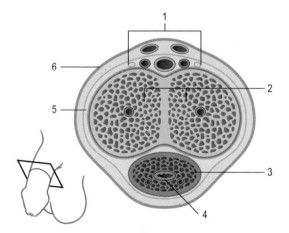

Fig 259

1. Blood vessels and nerves
2. Corpora cavernosa
3. Corpus spongiosum
4. Urethra
5. Connective tissue
6. Skin

Comments

Anatomical: The body of the penis is made up of two corpora cavernosa and one corpus spongiosum, which are erectile tissues that make erection possible. Two cylinders of erectile tissue constitute the corpora cavernosa, which surround the single centrally located corpus spongiosum, made up of spongy tissue. The external urethral meatus is located at the distal bulbous extremity of the penis, which consists of spongy tissue and is surrounded by the prepuce. The prepuce is a skin fold that covers the glans penis.

Physiological: These erectile bodies allow erection to occur.

Clinical: The combination of a decrease in the size and rigidity of the penis, failure to obtain and maintain an erection, testicular atrophy and psychological or neurological or vascular problems raises the possibility of erectile dysfunction. This condition is the inability to obtain and maintain an erection hard enough to allow vaginal penetration and leads to failure to achieve sexual satisfaction.

Section of the male reproductive organs

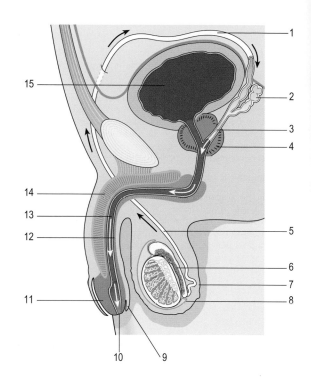

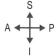

Fig 260

1. Vas deferens
2. Seminal vesicle
3. Ejaculatory duct
4. Prostate
5. Vas deferens in the spermatic cord
6. Epididymis
7. Scrotum
8. Testis
9. Prepuce
10. External urethral meatus
11. Glans penis
12. Corpus spongiosum
13. Urethra
14. Corpus cavernosum
15. Bladder

Comments

Anatomical: A mature spermatozoon is made up of a head, a body and a tail.

Physiological: Spermatozoa are made during spermatogenesis, which occurs in the testicular seminiferous tubules, and they undergo maturation in the epididymis. During ejaculation, they are expelled from the epididymis into the vas deferens and are then propelled through the ejaculatory duct, the urethra and the external urethral sphincter. The spermatozoa take 12 days, on average, to travel from the testis to the ejaculate. The mobility of the sperm depends on its tail or flagellum and the ability of its head to rotate 180 degrees.

Clinical: The process of spermatogenesis starts at puberty, on average between 12 and 14 years of age, as a result of hormonal stimulation. Spermatogenesis slows down at about 40 years of age but continues until the end of life.